Current Challenges with their Evolving Solutions in Surgical Practice in West Africa

A Reader

Editors

E.Q. Archampong

V.A. Essuman

J.C.B. Dakubo

J.N Clegg-Lamptey

DEPARTMENT OF SURGERY

**UNIVERSITY OF GHANA MEDICAL SCHOOL
COLLEGE OF HEALTH SCIENCES**

UNIVERSITY OF GHANA READERS

CLINICAL SCIENCES SERIES NO. 1

First published in Ghana 2013 for THE UNIVERSITY OF GHANA
by **Sub-Saharan Publishers**
P.O.Box 358
Legon-Accra
Ghana
Email: saharanp@africaonline.com.gh

© University of Ghana, 2013,
P.O.Box LG 25
Legon- Accra
Ghana
Tel: +233-302-500381
website:http://www.ug.edu.gh

ISBN:**978-9988-8602-2-6**

Contents

Contents

List of Tables

List of Figures

Foreword

The University of Ghana is celebrating sixty-five years of its founding this year. In all those years, lecturers and researchers of the university have contributed in quite significant ways to the development of thought and in the analyses of critical issues for Ghanaian and African societies. The celebration of the anniversary provides an appropriate opportunity for a reflection on the contributions that Legon academics have made to the intellectual development of Ghana and Africa. That is the aim of the University of Ghana Readers Project.

In the early years of the University, all the material that was used to teach students came largely from the United Kingdom and other parts of Europe. Most of the thinking in all disciplines was largely Eurocentric. The material that was used to teach students was mainly European, as indeed were many of the academics teaching the students. The norms and standards against which students were assessed were influenced largely by European values. The discussions that took place in seminar and lecture rooms were driven largely by what Africa could learn from Europe.

The 1960s saw a major 'revisionism' in African intellectual development as young African academics began to question received ideas against a backdrop of changing global attitudes in the wake of political independence. Much serious writing was done by African academics as their contribution to the search for new ways of organizing their societies. African intellectuals contributed to global debates in their own right and sometimes developed their own material for engaging with their students and the wider society.

Since the late 1970s universities in the region and their academics have struggled to make their voices heard in national and global debates. Against a new backdrop of economic stagnation and political disarray, many of the ideas for managing their economies and societies have come from outside. These ideas have often come with significant financial backing channelled through international organizations and governments. During the period, African governments saw themselves as having no reason to expect or ask for any intellectual contribution from their own academics. This was very much the case in Ghana.

The story is beginning to change in universities in many African countries. The University of Ghana Readers Project is an attempt to document the different ideas and debates that have influenced various disciplines over many years through collections of short essays and articles. They show the work of Legon academics and their collaborators in various disciplines as they have sought to introduce their research communities and students to new ideas. Our expectation is that this will mark a new beginning of solid engagement between Legon and other academics as they document their thoughts and contributions to the continuing search for new ideas to shape our world.

We gratefully acknowledge a generous grant from the Carnegie Corporation of New York that has made the publication of this series of Readers possible.

Ernest Aryeetey
Vice-Chancellor, University of Ghana.
Legon, August 2013

Preface

E.Q. Archampong

The Vice Chancellor's call to the various sections of the University for the publication of Readers resonates very well with the desires and aspirations of many senior members of the diverse sections of the College of Health Sciences. Some see this as an opportunity for dissemination of non-technical information on topical issues of general interest to the public, i.e. reinforcement of the public health education mission in the health sciences. Others, feeling that much has already transpired in this area, for example through the publication of books such as *The Layman's Guide to Good Health*[1] etc are inclined to explore the development of learning materials within their particular disciplines.

In the Department of Surgery several senior members were attracted to the latter idea, targeting learning materials for the ever increasing number of residents in the postgraduate programmes in the Department. Worldwide, there is a plethora of study materials in the form of authoritative review articles on disease entities afflicting the Western world but relatively few publications exploring similar problems confronting the developing countries, where resource limitation adds an extra dimension to the challenges facing the clinician.

The contributions received aim therefore to address common surgical challenges and what measures have evolved to overcome these problems. This Reader therefore addresses "Current Surgical Practice", placing emphasis on the principles underlying the consensus opinions prevailing in surgical management. The approach is practical, avoiding the minutiae of procedures by providing appropriate references detailing such information. The contributions address a broad swathe of critical management problems in the salient fields of surgery. Regrettably some urgent areas of public interest are not covered but it is clear that this volume represents the beginning of a process, indeed, the initiation of an epoch of Recent Advances in Surgical Practice. We are confident that this publication will stimulate further efforts to fill the yawning gaps in coverage.

This publication highlights developments in the prevention of childhood blindness in the country; global developments in premalignant and malignant disease of the breast are widely reviewed. The challenges in management of common disease entities such as acute appendicitis, peptic ulcer, and its complications, colorectal and gastric carcinoma, and emerging new patterns of neoplasia such as gastrointestinal stromal tumours (GIST). Some refreshing thoughts are expressed on old problems such as biliary tract and urinary tract obstruction. Departmental experience on fairly common challenges in infant care such as club foot and oesophageal atresia are reviewed. The development of one of the centres of excellence in the Department of Surgery, namely the National Cardiothoracic Centre is also highlighted.

References

1.   Health and Disease: A Layman's Guide to Good Health. (Eds). E.A. Badoe and S.K. Owusu. University of Ghana Medical / Smart Line Limited, Accra. 2011.

Contributors

1. **A.O. Addo MB, ChB, FRCS, FWACS, FGCS.**
   Senior Lecturer,
   Orthopaedic Surgery Unit,
   Department of Surgery,
   University of Ghana Medical School,
   College of Health Sciences,
   University of Ghana.
   Research interest: Joint diseases in patients with sickle cell disease.

2. **Nii Armah Adu-Aryee, MB.ChB, FWACS, FGCS.**
   Senior Lecturer,
   Department of Surgery,
   University of Ghana Medical School,
   College of Health Sciences,
   University of Ghana.
   Research interest: Genetics of gastric cancers in Africans.

3. **William Appeadu-Mensah, MB.ChB, BSc. (HB), FWACS, FGCS.**
   Lecturer,
   Paediatric Surgery Unit,
   Department of Surgery,
   University of Ghana Medical School,
   College of Health Sciences,
   University of Ghana.
   Research interest: Paediatric urology.

4. **E.Q. Archampong BSc, MS, FRCS, FWACS, FICS, FGCS, FGA, COV.**
   Emeritus Professor,
   Department of Surgery,
   University of Ghana Medical School,
   College of Health Sciences,

University of Ghana.
Research interest: Hepatic diseases; upper gastrointestinal
pathologies in Ghana.

5. **Ben Baako MB.ChB, FRCS, FWACS, FGCS.**
   Senior Lecturer,
   Department of Surgery,
   University of Ghana Medical School,
   College of Health Sciences,
   University of Ghana.
   Research interest: Surgical nutrition; breast cancer.

6. **K. Bandoh, MB. Ch.B, MRCS(Eng.), FWACS, FGCS.**
   Specialist,
   Orthopaedic Surgery Unit,
   Department of Surgery,
   Korle-Bu Teaching Hospital,
   Accra.
   Research interest: 1. Club foot corrections. 2. Shoulder arthroplasty
   and reconstruction.

7. **Joe Nat Clegg-Lamptey, MB.ChB, FRCS, FWACS, FGCS,**
   PgCBA.
   Associate Professor and Head of Department,
   Department of Surgery,
   University of Ghana Medical School,
   College of Health Sciences,
   University of Ghana.
   Research interest: 1. Breast cancer: Molecular and epidemiological
   characteristics in Ghana. 2. The vermiform appendix.

8. **Jonathan C.B. Dakubo, MB.ChB, FWACS, FGCS, BSc. (HB).**
   Senior Lecturer,
   Department of Surgery,
   University of Ghana Medical School,
   College of Health Sciences,

University of Ghana.
Research interest: Genetics and epidemiology of colorectal cancers in Africans.

9. **Rudolph Darko, MB.ChB, FRCS, FWACS, FGCS, FICS, MOV.**
   Associate Professor,
   Department of Surgery,
   University of Ghana Medical School,
   College of Health Sciences,
   University of Ghana.
   Research interest: Hepatobiliary diseases in Ghana, emphasis on gallstone disease.

10. **Florence Dedey, MB ChB, FWACS,**
    Lecturer,
    Department of Surgery,
    University of Ghana Medical School,
    College of Health Sciences,
    University of Ghana.
    Research interest: Breast diseases.

11. **Vera Adobea Essuman, MB ChB, FWACS, FGCS.**
    Senior Lecturer/ Paediatric Ophthalmologist
    Ophthalmology Unit,
    Department of Surgery,
    University of Ghana Medical School, College of Health Sciences,
    University of Ghana.
    Research interest: Epidemiology and therapeutic interventions for major causes of childhood blindness.

12. **K. Frimpong-Boateng, MB, ChB, FWACS, FGCS, FGA MD, FA Chirug; Arzt Thorax und Kardiovasc Chirug.; Arzt Gaefass Chirug.**
    Professor,
    Cardiothoracic Surgery Unit,

Department of Surgery,
University of Ghana Medical School,
College of Health Sciences,
University of Ghana.
Research interest: Cardiothoracic disorders.

13. **E.D. Kitcher, MB.ChB, FRCS, FWACS, FGCS.**
Senior Lecturer,
Ear, Nose & Throat Unit (ENT),
Department of Surgery,
University of Ghana Medical School,
College of Health Sciences,
University of Ghana.
Research interest: Noise and its effect on hearing

14. **Mathew Y. Kyei, MB.ChB, FWACS.**
Lecturer,
Urology Unit,
Department of Surgery,
University of Ghana Medical School,
College of Health Sciences,
University of Ghana.
Research interest: Urology, oncology, especially prostate cancers.

15. **Simon B. Naaeder, MB.ChB, MD (UG), FRCS, FWACS, FGCS.**
Professor,
Department of Surgery,
University of Ghana Medical School,
College of Health Sciences,
University of Ghana.
Research interest: Colorectal diseases.

16. **Michael Segbefia, MB. ChB, FWACS.**
Lecturer,
Orthopaedic Surgery Unit,

Department of Surgery,
University of Ghana Medical School,
College of Health Sciences,
University of Ghana.
Research interest: Paediatric orthopaedics: deformity correction, limb lengthening, spine diseases.

17. **Verna Vandepuye, MB.ChB, FWACS, FGCS, BSc. (HB).**
National Radiotherapy Centre
Korle-Bu.
Part-Time Lecturer,
School of Allied Health Sciences,
College of Health Sciences,
University of Ghana.
Research interest: Chemoradiotherapy; breast cancers and gynaecological cancers.

Chapter 1
Department of Surgery Profile

J. N. Clegg-Lamptey

The Department of Surgery was one of the first Departments established in the University of Ghana Medical School. The Clinical Department currently spans the main six-storey Surgical Block, Cardiothoracic Centre, National Burns Plastic and Reconstruction centre, Accident Centre and Allied Surgery wards of the Korle Bu Teaching Hospital.

It is arguably the largest department in the University of Ghana, with a teaching staff strength of 49. The Department boasts a unique blend of many generations of teachers. They include some of the pioneers who established the Department (Professors E. A. Badoe and E.Q. Archampong) and others such as Dr. B. A. Kuma and Prof. E. D. Yeboah who have taught for many decades and trained generations of teachers and students. Their rich experience and dedication combined with the youthful dynamism and technological savvy of some of the very young teachers have greatly enriched the Department.

Some past senior members have put Ghana on the world map through their innovations and achievements. They include Prof. Kwashie Quartey (who introduced the Quartey Urethroplasty operation), Prof. E. A. Badoe (Badoe intravenous fluid) and Prof. Frimpong-Boateng (First black African to carry out heart transplantation).

Starting off with General Surgery, the Department has expanded into nine units that are currently striving to subspecialize:

1. General Surgery,
2. Plastic Surgery,
3. Trauma and Orthopaedic Surgery,
4. Urology,
5. Neurosurgery,
6. Cardiothoracic Surgery,
7. Paediatric Surgery,
8. Ophthalmology,
9. Ear, Nose and Throat surgery.

The first Head of the Department was Professor Charles Easmon (in 1966) who also served as the first Dean of the Medical School. The Department has since had many illustrious heads:

Prof. C. O. Easmon	1 January 1966 – 31 December 1971
Prof. E. A. Badoe	1 January 1972 – 31March 1981
Prof. E. Q. Archampong	1 April 1981 – 31 March 1990
Prof. E. D. Yeboah	1 April 1990 – 30 September 1997
Prof. S. B. Naaeder	1 October 1997 – 31 December 2000
Prof. K. Frimpong-Boateng	1 January 2001 – 31 August 2002
Prof. R. Darko	1 September 2002 – 31 July 2008
Prof. A. A .J. Hesse	1 August 2008 – 31 July 2010
Prof. J. N. Clegg-Lamptey	1 August 2010 - Present

Core Functions

1. Teaching/ Training

The Department offers teaching and training of medical students in the University of Ghana Medical School during the three clinical years:

First Clinical Year

General Surgery, Paediatric Surgery, Urology, Neurosurgery, Orthopaedics & Trauma:

Second Clinical Year

ENT, Ophthalmology.

Third Clinical Year

General Surgery, Paediatric Surgery, Cardiothoracic Surgery, Plastic Surgery, Orthopaedic Surgery, Neurosurgery, Urology.

We also offer training to students from other Schools and Postgraduate colleges:

- Dental students from the University of Ghana Dental School;
- Nursing students from School of Nursing;

- Postgraduate surgical trainees of the Ghana College of Physicians and Surgeons and the West African College of Surgeons;
- Foreign medical students on Exchange and Elective programmes;
- Foreign-trained doctors, in preparation for Ghana Medical & Dental Council examinations;
- House officers and nursing interns.

2. Service

The Department provides specialist consultancy and theatre services for referred surgical cases from all over the country and the West African subregion. Many senior members go on outreach programmes to various parts of the country, and some offer weekly breast screening to the public in the Korle Bu Teaching hospital.

3. Research

The Department undertakes research in all its specialties and also does collaborative research with other institutions such as the University of Ghana, Ministry of Health, and external agencies.

There is an active monthly Research Forum that promotes research in the department.

Future Directions

Teaching sites

With the forthcoming relocation of the College of Health Sciences to Legon campus, the Department envisages that it will soon be operating from two main sites (Legon and Korle Bu) as well as the Military Hospital. We will explore the possibility of additional sites so that medical students can be taught more effectively in the light of increasing student numbers.

Manpower development

More strenuous efforts at recruiting young faculty will continue. The Department hopes to have young faculty in every unit who are motivated to develop their specialties.

Young faculty will be trained in Israel under the programme to build a new Teaching Hospital at the Legon campus. We will also look for other avenues for young specialists to spend some time in highly specialized centres overseas in order to encourage sub-specialization.

Academic degrees

Senior members will actively encourage young specialists to aim at academic degrees (e.g. MD, PhD) soon after their fellowship examinations.

Research

There will be strengthening of the Department's Research Forum, where research topics are discussed and useful suggestions given. Other measures to encourage senior members and residents to conduct research will be implemented.

Young faculty will also be supported to study and become proficient in research methods through activities like the Cardiovascular Research Training (CART) programme.

E-Learning and innovations in teaching

The Department will continue to explore new and efficient ways of teaching and examination. This will include e-learning and other innovative teaching methods. OSCE will continue and be further evaluated for possible use at the final MB ChB examination.

Chapter 2
The World through the Child's Eyes –
The Journey Towards Elimination of Childhood
Blindness in Ghana – The Korle-Bu Experience

V. A. Essuman

Introduction
Childhood Blindness Worldwide
UNICEF (United Nations Children's Fund or originally the *United Nations International Children's Emergency Fund*) defines a child as an individual aged less than 16 years. The World Health Organisation (WHO) defines blindness as a corrected visual acuity in the better eye of less than 3/60, and severe visual impairment as a corrected acuity in the better eye of less than 6/60.[1]

It is estimated that every-minute a child goes blind in the world – an estimated 500,000 new cases per year[1]. The prevalence of blindness in children varies according to the socioeconomic development and under-5 mortality rates. In low-income countries with high under-5 mortality rates, the prevalence may be as high as 1.5 per 1000 children, while in high-income countries with low under-5 mortality rates, the prevalence is around 0.3 per 1000 children.[2] Most of these children will live in poverty. Three quarters of the world's blind children live in the developing world and about half of the cases the causes of their blindness are avoidable (i.e. preventable or treatable).

More than 50 per cent will die within 1-2 years of going blind. Those children who do survive with blindness, an estimated 1.4 million worldwide, then have an entire life of visual impairment before them.[1,3]

Taking these 'blind years' into account, the scale of blindness in children is second only to cataract as a global cause of blindness – an estimated 70 million blind years.[3]

Childhood Blindness in Ghana

The elimination of preventable and treatable causes of childhood visual disability is a priority for intervention in Ghana. The prevalence of blindness in children, 0-15 years old, is estimated to be 0.9 per 1,000 children. Most causes of childhood blindness in Ghana are avoidable.[4,5,6]

History of WHO/Lions Club International/ Government of Ghana Project for the Elimination of Childhood Blindness in Ghana

The World Health Organization (WHO) has identified the prevention, treatment and control of blindness and visual impairment in childhood as a priority area of work. Childhood blindness is one of the major causes of avoidable blindness worldwide and thus targeted under the Vision 2020 Initiative for the Elimination of Avoidable Blindness[1]

In June 2003, WHO launched the five-year (2003-2007) childhood blindness prevention project. Centres for comprehensive children's eye care and low-vision care were established in 30 countries, including Ghana. The Korle Bu Teaching Hospital (KBTH) in the Greater Accra Region, was the centre of the Ghana project covering the Greater Accra and Eastern regions of the country (Figure 1) with a population of 5,200,000 [children < 15 years = 2.2 million]. A model Child Friendly Eye Care Centre (CFECC) was thus established in KBTH to serve this population in particular and the whole country generally. The project was further extended under a Bridge Grant [2008-2011], Ghana being one of 25 countries [out of the initial 30 countries] to benefit from the extension. This model is to be replicated later in the country.

The project was supported financially by the Lions Clubs International, through the Sight First Programme of the Lion Clubs International Foundation (LCIF), with the WHO (Prevention of Blindness and Deafness) as the Executing Agency, in partnership with the Ghana Government.

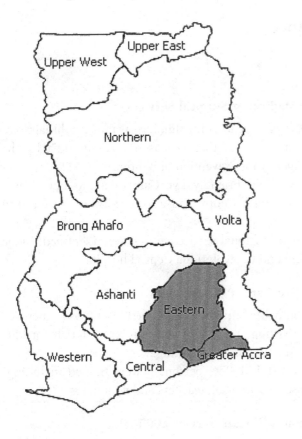

Figure 2.1: Project area

Goal and Objectives for the Project

- **Goal**
  - Eliminate avoidable childhood blindness in Ghana
- **Specific objectives:**
  - to provide Primary Eye Care (PEC) in PHC;
  - to develop surgical/medical paediatric Eye Care Service (ECS);
  - to establish/strengthen Low Vision Service (LVS);
  - to develop & strengthen infrastructure & equipment;
  - to conduct monitoring and evaluation of project.

A. Performance

I. Training

i. Paediatric Medical & Surgical Services

In 2003/2004, a paediatric ophthalmology team (2 ophthalmologists, 1 nurse and 1 anaesthetist) was trained in India by the International Agency for Prevention of Blindness - (IAPB)

In July 2004, a Child Friendly Eye Care Centre (CFECC) was established as a Service Centre and also as a Training Centre in Korle-Bu.

In 2005, two extra regional service centres were identified: Ridge hospital in Accra and the Koforidua Central hospital.

ii. Primary Eye Care (PEC) Services

In 2005, 20 ophthalmic nurses were trained in PEC as trainers for PEC workers. Existing curriculum and training materials for PEC were reviewed and adapted for training.

In the same year 1,154 PEC personnel were trained including-community-based health staff, teachers and volunteers.

iii. Low Vision (LV) Care Service 2005/2006

In 2005/2006, the following were achieved for low vision care:

- A team was trained, made up of one ophthalmologist as trainer in Hong Kong and two optometrists in Pakistan and South Africa.
- The low vision team at the CFECC provided training by orienting in LV care 3 ophthalmologists, 4 optometrists, 4 ophthalmic nurses, 4 teachers and 1 low vision client to work in the project area.
- Four ophthalmic nurses were fully trained locally in LV care.
- LV Centres were established in KBTH and Koforidua Regional Hospital.

II. Infrastructure and Equipment at the CFECC

- A LV clinic and LV equipment were in place by 2005/2006 at KBTH.
- Provision of basic equipment and instruments for paediatric medical and surgical care at the CFECC continued throughout the project period.
- A child-friendly play area and a library of books were established at the Outpatient clinic of the CFECC in 2009-2010. This was through the support of parents/guardians, private individuals and corporate bodies (Figure 2.2).

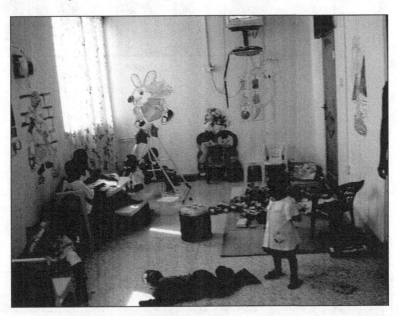

Figure 2.2: Children's play area at the CFECC, KBTH.

III. Service Delivery

i.   There has been a progressive increase in out-patient attendance at the CFECC (Figure 2.3).

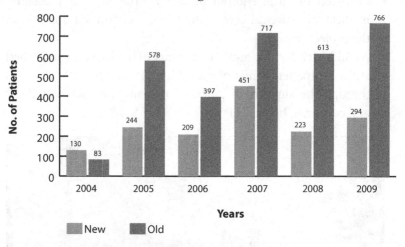

Figure 2.3: Out-patient attendance at the CFECC, KBTH

ii.   New diseases continue to be seen at the Outpatient Clinic of the CFECC, KBTH, including major causes of avoidable blindness (Table 2.1).

| Table 2.1 | Service Delivery - Yearly Summary of Top Seven New Diseases (CFECC- KORLE BU) | | | | | | |

Disease	2004	2005	2006	2007	2008	2009	Total
Cataract	12	41	101	56	31	48	289
Conjunctivitis	30	108	37	18	8	5	206
Strabismus	14	19	16	39	36	40	164
Glaucoma	6	7	24	33	6	30	106
Refractive error	12	24	8	19	6	0	69
Retinoblastoma	8	15	5	10	9	13	60
Cornea /Ant. Seg.	8	14	2	5	11	6	46
Others	40	16	16	271	116	152	611
Total	130	244	209	451	223	294	1551

iii. Causes of Childhood Blindness at Korle Bu Teaching Hospital

Bilateral Causes	Unilateral Causes
Cataract	Retinoblastoma
Glaucoma	Cataract
Cortical visual impairment	Injuries- Broomstick
Refractive error	Others
Cornea/Vernalkerato-conjunctivitis	
Others	

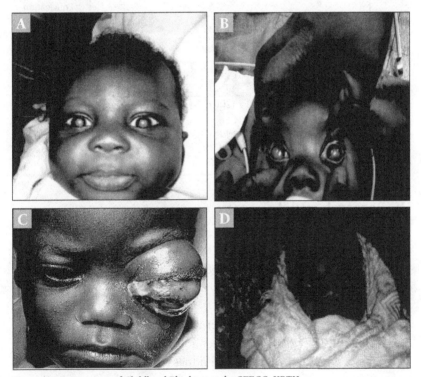

Figure 2.4: Some causes of Childhood Blindness at the CFECC, KBTH
A- Bilateral Congenital Cataract – opacity of the lens
B- Congenital Glaucoma
C - Retinoblastoma – Cancer of the retina
D- Ophthalmia neonatorum

Specialised paediatric eye surgeries are now performed (Figure 2.5) with better outcomes. However, only about half the number of children requiring surgeries receive this treatment. The most important reason for this under performance is the inadequate provision of general anaesthesia due to lack of a dedicated anaesthetist for paediatric eye surgical procedures.

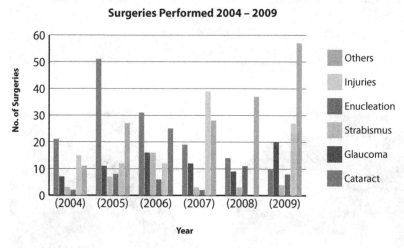

Figure 2.5: Surgeries performed at the CFECC, KBTH.

IV. Research and Advocacy

The following have either been achieved or are ongoing in this category of performance:
- Scientific presentations at both local and international fora;
- Public lectures;
- Radio & television talks;
- Scientific publications in peer-reviewed journals.[7,8]
- Ongoing research into epidemiological and clinical trials for major causes of childhood blindness in Ghana.
- A fund to cater for the treatment of the needy but blind children and also for the acquisition of equipment, instruments and consummables, has been in existence since 2007 through the advocacy of the team at the CFECC. This fund for the control of childhood blindness depends on the generous support of

private individuals, parents/ guardians, establishments and corporate bodies. The fund is managed by the University of Ghana Medical School.

Strengths, Weaknesses, Opportunities and Threats (SWOT) Analysis of the Project

The childhood blindness prevention can further point to significant accomplishments and strengths such as the recognition of the centre/ project in Ghana and in neighbouring countries (Togo, Ivory-coast, Liberia and Sierra Leone) resulting in the centre receiving referrals from all over the country and also from these neighbouring countries. In addition, the country now has access to specialised paediatric medical, surgical and low vision services, augmented by the dedicated eye theatre at the CFECC, KBTH.

The gains of the project are further highlighted by the incorpo-ration of Child Eye Health into the curricula of residency programmes in ophthalmology (West African College of Surgeons, Ghana College of Physicians and Surgeons) and Ophthalmic Nurses Training School at (KBTH). Thus, cadres of the eye care are being progressively trained for the elimination of childhood blindness throughout the country.

The establishment of the National Task Team in 2005, an oversight body for the Elimination of Childhood Blindness especially by CFECC, gave the project further impetus. The task team draws representatives from: Local Lions Club, National School Health Programme, Ministry of Women & Children's Affairs, Integrated Management of Childhood Illness[IMCI], WHO, Ghana Health Service, Society of Paediatricians, National Eye Care Programme and a Paediatric Ophthalmologist from the CFECC. The team is presently inactive but is expected to resume its role with the start of the Phase 2 of the project later in 2013.

Over the years, the CFECC has had its share of weaknesses that threaten to undermine its progress, including the late presen-tation of children with blinding conditions such as retinoblastoma[7], congenital glaucoma[8] and congenital cataracts. Compounding this are the inadequate provision of general anaesthesia coverage resulting in fewer surgeries performed; irregular supplies of surgical instruments and consumables such as intraocular lenses, vitrector probes and affordable spectacles; poor reporting systems and data management among others.

Sustaining the gains of CFECC activities in particular and the project as a whole, will require pragmatic steps. These should include health education of the general public and health professionals on these conditions, early detection and funding for treatment. There are on-going research projects to find out the reasons for the late presentations of some of the major causes of childhood blindness at the CFECC.

Another aspect of the CFECC's quest to eliminate childhood blindness in Ghana is the establishment of the Moorfields Eye Hospital Foundation Surgical Training Centre for West Africa in KBTH which is expected to be completed in the year 2013. This collaboration between Moorfields Eye Hospital (UK) and the West African College of Surgeons will include a paediatric wing with out-patient, play area and in-patient care. There will also be an opportunity for subspecialty/ fellowship training in paediatric ophthalmology and other eyecare workers.

As regards funding for treatment, the establishment of the National Health Insurance Scheme by the government and the Fund for the Needy and Blind Children, spearheaded by the CFECC team are helping greatly. However more donors are needed for this cause.

There is a dedicated computer for data management. There is the need however, for a dedicated data management clerk. Ultimately, the computerisation of the KBTH hospital medical records system would improve on data management.

Low-vision service in the country has also been further enhanced by the care provision and human resource development supported by Sight Savers International (SSI) in two regions for the pilot project in Phase 1. The establishment of integrated schools for visually challenged children in Ghana by the Government with additional support from Force Foundation (Netherlands), through the supply of LV aids (e.g. CCTV, braille and vision assessment tools to universities, integrated second cycle schools and schools for the visually challenged) continue to impact greatly on the elimination of visual impairment in Ghanaian children.

The ongoing establishment of a second Paediatric Ophthalmology Centre at Komfo Anokye Teaching Hospital, Kumasi, to cater for the northern sector of the country is an added advantage.

The support for comprehensive primary eye care in the project area by Sight Savers International and in the two Northern regions (Action Against Childhood Blindness, AACHIB) by Swiss Red Cross, further demonstrates the important role and partnership that non-governmental development organisations provide in the country's effort to eliminate childhood blindness and improve on the general eye health of Ghanaian children.

However, the success of the CFECC is threatened by the erratic supply of equipment and consummables by KBTH. In addition, the inadequate provision of general anaesthesia has been one of the major threats to the success of the project.

Going Forward/ Future Plans

Phase 2 of the WHO/Lions Club International/ Government of Ghana Project for the Elimination of Childhood Blindness. In January 2011 the SightFirst Advisory Committee (SAC) of the LCIF approved a two-year extension [2012- 2014] of the project for 10 of the best-performing institutions worldwide. The CFECC, thanks to its previous success, was chosen to receive funding in order to upgrade the existing CFECC at the Korle Bu Teaching Hospital, to create a new satellite center at the Ga South Municipal Hospital in Weija, and to support the training of local staff in the areas of primary eye care and paediatric surgery.

Training of practising ophthalmologists to augment skills in medical and surgical care in paediatric eye health; fellowship training in paediatric ophthalmology and the establishment of low-vision teams for other regions will continue to engage the centre's attention.

The increasing numbers of children with eye health needs attending the CFECC have brought to the fore the need to **establish a Counselling Unit** for patients and parents/ carers at the centre to enhance patient and carer education and also free the doctors to dedicate their time and efforts to the medical and surgical care of the children.

Efforts will be made to strengthen the referral systems and collaboration with other stakeholders in the Elimination of Childhood Blindness locally, especially with the new unit at KATH and with all the peripheral eye clinics in the country.

Finally, attention will be given to collaboration with external and local institutions in the area of mentorship programmes and in research.

Conclusion

This pilot project for the elimination of childhood blindness in Ghana has been a good programme in spite of the teething challenges. There is the need for more advocacy and additional sourcing of funding to ensure sustainability of the project. Finally, it will be important to continue with the building of strong teams and fostering multi-sectoral and collaborative linkages both locally and internationally.

Appreciation/Acknowledgements

Special appreciation to the following:
   i.   LICF-SF / WHO;
   ii. Govt. of Ghana – GHS, MOH, University of Ghana Medical School;
   iii. All other partners: Sight Savers International, Swiss Red Cross, Operation Eyesight Universal;
   iv. Task Team for the Elimination of Childhood Blindness in Ghana.

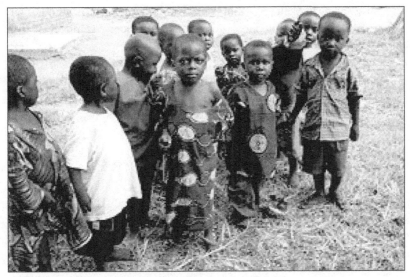

Figure 2.6: Keep our children's eyes healthy, for they are our future.

References

1. Gilbert, C., Foster, A. Childhood blindness in the context of VISION 2020- The Right to Sight. Bulletin of the World Health Organization, 2001, 79: 227–232.
2. Gilbert C.E., Anderton, L., Dandona, L. Foster, A. Prevalence of visual impairment in children: A review of available data. *Ophthalmic Epidemiology. 1999, 6:73-82.*
3. World Health Organization. Preventing blindness in children -www. who.int/ncd/vision2020_actionplan/.../WHO_PBL_00.77
4. Akafo, S. K. and Hagan, M. Causes of childhood blindness in Southern Ghana–a blind school survey, *Ghana Med J,* 1990; 24:113-9.
5. Ntim-Amponsah, C.T and Amoaku, W.M.K., Causes of Visual Impairment and Unmet Low Vision Care in a School for the Blind, *Int Ophthalmol,* 2008; 28:317–23.
6. Gyasi, M.E. Setting the pace for Vision 2020 in Ghana: the case of Bawku Eye Care Program, *Community Eye Health,* 2006; 19(59):46–7.

7.   Essuman, V, Akafo, S., Ntim-Amponsah, C.T., Renner, L., and Edusei
      L. Presentation of Retinoblastoma at a Paediatric Eye Clinic in Ghana.
      Ghana Medical Journal. 2010; 44:10-15.
8.   Essuman V. A., Braimah I. Z., Ndanu T. A. and Ntim-Amponsah, C. T.
      Combined trabeculotomy and trabeculectomy: outcome for primary
      congenital glaucoma in a West African population. *Eye*.201125:
      77–83; doi:10.1038/eye.2010.156; published online 5 November
      2010.

Chapter 3
Current Global Developments in Breast Cancer and Management in Ghana

J. N. Clegg-Lamptey and V. Vanderpuye

Introduction

Breast cancer is the leading female malignancy in the world with about one million new cases diagnosed annually, over 400,000 annual deaths and about 4.4 million women living with the disease.[1] In Ghana it is one of the leading cancers in all institutional data, constituting 16 percent of all cancers from the pathology records of the Korle Bu Teaching hospital and 28 percent of presenting cases at the Radiotherapy Centre of the same hospital. The management of the disease is however continually changing and it is necessary to alter management strategies from time to time in the light of current clinical evidence.

In this chapter we will look at some of the current developments and trends in breast cancer management. We will also discuss some established current practice that, in our view, is not yet manifest in our practice in Ghana.

General developments

a. Multidisciplinary team work

Breast cancer used to be managed solely by the surgeon whose word was final. Currently this method is outmoded. Management decisions are now so complex, taking into consideration a variety of factors and involving other specialties, that it is not advisable to leave them in the hands of a single decision maker including the physician.

It is now widely accepted that multidisciplinary teams (MDTs) form the basis for best practice in the management of breast disease.[2] Multidisciplinary team work was appropriately the first key recommendation of the National Institute for Clinical Excellence (NICE) in the United Kingdom.[3] Their recommendations were as follows:

- All patients with breast cancer should be managed by multidisciplinary teams and all multidisciplinary teams should be actively involved in network-wide audit of processes and outcomes.
- Multidisciplinary teams should consider how they might improve the effectiveness of the way they work.

The recommended team is made up of all key players in the patient's management, namely the surgeon, breast care nurse, pathologist, radiologist, radiation oncologist, medical oncologist, psychologist, clinical pharmacist, plastic/reconstruction surgeon and the social worker. Other specialties may form part of the team based on local circumstances: a clinical psychologist and clinical pharmacist play a very important role in the breast MDT at the Korle Bu Teaching Hospital. Patients should be considered members of the team and their views considered in arriving at management decisions. The guidelines by the Association of Breast Surgery, Royal College of Surgeons of England suggest two teams, a diagnostic team and a management team[2]

In the Korle Bu Teaching Hospital, a MDT runs a 'Breast Clinic' every Tuesday. A tumour board is also run at the Komfo Anokye Teaching Hospital. These teams discuss patients with breast cancer and reach consensus about treatment. Often patients are brought to the meeting, examined and discussed.

b. Patient -centred care

Breast cancer is a heterogeneous disease and management should be individualized, taking the circumstances of each patient into consideration. Many factors, including the pathology of the disease, stage and quality of life issues have to be considered. In developing countries, the availability of resources and sometimes the high cost of some forms of treatment influence management decisions to a large extent[4].

c. Use of protocols

To prevent arbitrariness, agreed protocols should guide patient management. Protocols should be based on current global clinical evidence, evidence from local practice, peculiarities of local practice and any on-going clinical trials as this will most likely lead to optimal outcomes[5].

d. Clinical trials

Breast units are encouraged to support clinical research and are expected to participate in multicentre studies aimed at improving treatment for breast cancer. There is some evidence that patients treated in clinical trials have improved outcomes.[6] In spite of difficulties in obtaining funding for research, developing countries need to carry out clinical trials of their own. This is because genetic, social, demographic, environmental, and geographic attributes affect outcomes across countries and communities.[7]

Diagnosis of breast cancer

a. Current developments in screening:

Screening for cancer has become a standard of practice in contemporary health care.[8] Mammographic screening has been shown to be effective. Indeed, the Cochrane 2006 report estimates a 15percent relative risk reduction following mammographic screening.[9] Breast -self examination has, however, not been found to have a similar benefit in reducing mortality from breast cancer.[10] The current recommendations are biennial screening mammography for women aged 50 to 74 years.[11]

There is no national screening programme in Ghana and many similar poorly resourced countries. Nonetheless, it is doubtful if a mammographic screening programme would have the same effect it has had in Western countries, since the majority of breast cancer patients in this country are young and the majority do not have access to mammography. Most of the patients report with advanced disease and after long periods of noticing breast abnormality. The problem therefore seems to be reluctance in seeking treatment. A principal goal in poorly resourced countries therefore should be "earlier detection to downstage symptomatic disease by teaching women the importance of seeking timely evaluation of breast symptoms"[12] .

In Ghana, breast cancer advocacy groups and groups of doctors and nurses sometimes organise talks and offer clinical breast examination, and encourage women to do breast self- examination. There is however no co-ordinated effort by the Ministry of Health to tackle the issue of screening/early detection.

The schedule below, recommended by the American Cancer Society and Susan Komen Breast Cancer foundation[13], is modified and can be implemented in Ghana in place of a national screening programme.

Breast Self-Examination (BSE)	Monthly	From Age 20
Clinical Breast Examination (CBE)	3 yearly	From Age 20
	then Yearly	From Age 40
Mammograms	Bi-anually	From Age 40
Women at increased risk:	Screen at earlier age, anually and use more accurate methods.	

We favour opportunistic mammographic screening rather than the creation of a national mammographic screening programme. Teaching women breast self-examination and the importance of timely intervention should be a priority whenever clinicians see their female patients.

b. Making screening more accurate:

Magnetic resonance imaging (MRI) and digital mammography are two sensitive imaging methods that can be used to detect early breast cancer[14]. Though they are more expensive than film mammography, they are more sensitive and make image storage easier. They are superior in detecting early breast cancer in pre- menopausal women, women under 50 and those with dense breasts. There is no advantage in using digital mammography in older, post-menopausal women. We must state that the expertise of the operator is also very important. The ultrasound has been found to be a vital tool when combined with mammography to improve accuracy, however on its own, it is not a recommended tool[15]. Cost constraint is one of the major hindrances to appropriate choice of screening method.

c. Triple Assessment

   i.   Clinical examination,

   ii.   Radiological assessment:

       Mammography,

       Ultrasonography,

       MRI,

       Digital mammography,

   iii.   Pathology (& cytology).

Triple assessment remains the means through which diagnosis of breast cancer is made.

In practice it works thus: patients are first evaluated clinically and radiologically. The results are discussed by the MDT. If both are negative there is no need for a biopsy. If one is suspicious or positive for carcinoma a biopsy is done.

Methods of taking biopsy (or cytology) include:

       Stereotactic biopsies,

       Ultrasound-guided biopsies,

       Wire localisation biopsies,

       Fine needle aspiration cytology (FNAC),

       Core biopsy,

       Incision biopsy,

       Excision biopsy.

Ultrasound guidance improves the accuracy of biopsy of palpable lesions. Stereotactic, image-guided and wire localisation biopsies are presently not offered by radiologists in our practice. These methods are needed to biopsy impalpable lesions detected on radiological assessment. As impalpable lesions are increasingly picked up by imaging techniques (like mammography and MRI) in Ghana, it has become necessary to develop these methods of biopsy.

As much as possible FNAC or core biopsies should be performed in obtaining tissue, rather than excision biopsy. However, very small lesions may be best excised. Incision biopsy is only indicated in ulcerated lesions, Pagets disease of the nipple and inflammatory breast cancer without a mass. If FNAC and core biopsies are equivocal open biopsy becomes necessary.

Pathology reports

To be useful for subsequent management decisions biopsy reports should include all the following details[16]:
Cell morphology including location;
>   Grading: 1, 2 or 3;
>   Lymphatic invasion;
>   Vascular invasion;
>   In situ components and proportions;
>   Size;
>   Margins (distance of tumour from the resection margins);
>   ER, PR receptor status and intensity of positivity;
>   HER-2 status.

Other important information that may be provided by the pathologist [17] but not available in Ghana include:

S phase fraction,
Ki 67,
Oncotype DX,
MammaPrint.
These additional tests help determine the aggressive nature of disease.

Treatment

The general principles of oncological treatments have not changed. Treatment is directed at the breast (surgery and/or radiotherapy), the axilla (surgery and/or radiotherapy) and the whole body (chemotherapy and/or hormonal therapy and/or biologic therapy). However, the sequence of modalities depends on various factors including the stage and, unique to us, availability of treatment and financial state of patient.

We will now discuss some aspects of surgery, hormonal therapy, chemotherapy and radiotherapy.

Surgical options I: Breast

Mastectomy has been practiced for many years, and is still the main operation performed in Ghana because most tumours are advanced. It is almost always done in combination with an axillary dissection.

There is a move towards breast conservation surgery with radiotherapy to the remaining breast in early breast cancer. This is called breast conservation (wide excision, lumpectomy, quadrantectomy, partial mastectomy). Much Level 1 evidence has shown that breast conservation treatment, when appropriately done, is comparable to mastectomy in early breast cancer[18]. The lump must be small, with 5cm actual maximum diameter, unifocal/unicentric, with no skin involvement as per most international guidelines. Slightly bigger and borderline tumours can be down-staged by neoadjuvant chemotherapy and the breast conserved if there is appropriate response.[19] There are contraindications to breast conservation such as persistent positive margin, connective tissue disease, large unresectable disease, recurrent disease and previous regional irradiation.[20] An acceptable margin of resection is 2mm. Re-excision is recommended if the margin is less as positive or close margins influence recurrence.[21]

Breast reconstruction is increasingly being undertaken by plastic surgeons and breast surgeons worldwide, using any of the following techniques alone or in combination: Implant (saline or gel) or autologous flap (Latissimus Dorsi [LD] or Tranverse rectus abdominis myocutaneous [TRAM]) and nipple reconstruction using tattoo and/or skin.[22] In Ghana, reconstruction is done in very few instances especially, with young women as there are few plastic surgeons in the country and it is very time consuming.

The range of surgical procedures for the breast can be summarised as:
- Breast conservation surgery (Wide excision, lumpectomy, quadrantectomy, etc);
- Re-excision surgery;
- Modified Radical Mastectomy (Mastectomy with axillary dissection);
- Breast reconstruction; Immediate or Delayed;
  - Implant (saline or gel);
  - Autologous flap (LD or TRAM);

- Flap + Implant;
- Nipple reconstruction: tattoo and/or skin;
- With contralateral breast reduction, etc.

Surgical options II: Axillary dissection

Axillary dissection or sampling is important for staging, prognosis and treatment[23]. Levels of axillary lymph nodes are defined by their relation to the pectoralis minor muscle. The choice of axillary exploration employed has to be selected for optimum benefit. These are:

Sentinel node biopsy,

4 node sampling,

Axillary Clearance: Level I [lower], II [middle] or III [apical].

Sentinel node biopsy[24] offers the chance for very minimal dissection and can be done under local anaesthesia if being done alone. It involves the use of a blue dye and/or radioactive tracer that is picked up by the first echelon of draining lymph nodes from the breast. The dyed or radioactive nodes are dissected and examined under frozen section for metastases. If positive in more than one, a full axillary dissection is employed. Recently, though, the American College of Surgeons' Z0011 study has raised issues regarding the value of full dissection following sentinel node biopsy in very early breast cancer.[25]

In Ghana, most patients have Level 1 and II axillary clearance because of the absence of logistics and expertise in implementation of sentinel node biopsy. Also, the underdevelopment of the technique is due to the fact that most breast cancer patients have axillary node involvement (about 70 per cent of breast cancer patients present with locally advanced disease)[26] and therefore most patients do not qualify for it. Level 111 clearance is known to cause the most complications and is not routinely performed unless they are seen to be involved during surgery.

The minimum recommended number of nodes for adequate prognostic evaluation after axillary clearance is six to ten nodes[27]. The percentage of involved node is now an acceptable alternative to prognostic evaluation of lymph node involvement.

There are very few instances in which axillary exploration can be exempt: carcinoma *in situ* and Pagets disease of nipple without a palpable lump.

Chemotherapy

This involves the use of cytotoxic and cytostatic drugs to manage breast cancer. The choice of drugs and sequencing have been established through various randomised studies[28]

Chemotherapy is usually given as a combination of drugs in the curative setting for at least four cycles but mostly an average of six cycles. Single- agent first line treatment is not recommended unless it is a continuation of a protocol or in the metastatic setting or as second-line therapy. It can be given before surgery (neoadjuvant) to make tumour resectable (Fig 3.1), or after surgery (adjuvant) to mop up or slow down possible circulating disease. Chemotherapy is used as monotherapy in the metastastic setting.

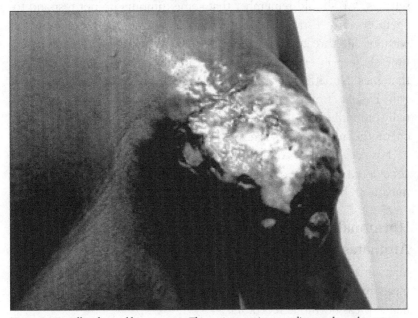

Figure 3.1: Locally advanced breast cancer. This patient requires neoadjuvant chemotherapy

It is important to assess response to chemotherapy in the neoadjuvant and palliative setting. This may warrant changing of medication for non-response or toxicity.

There are various combinations that include anthracyclines, 5-flourouracil, cyclophosphamide, methotrexate, taxanes, vinca alkaloids, pyrimidines, and platinums.[29] Each drug has specific toxicities which, if not monitored, could be life threatening. The most recognised and worrisome toxicity is cardiac morbidity leading to early death. Patients with pre-existing cardiac disease are at higher risk of added toxicity especially with the addition of chest wall irradiation. Causative drugs are anthracyclines, taxanes, flouropyrimidines and platinums. Some drugs such as the anthracyclines have lifetime dose limits (i.e. $400mg/m^2$) that should not be exceeded under any circumstance.[30]

New and novel chemotherapy drugs have improved the outcome of breast cancer over the last decade and could be applied in our settings. We should remember that some tumours do not respond to chemotherapy. Patients who are strongly hormone receptor-positive without life-threatening symptoms may not require chemotherapy unless there is evidence of progression after sequential hormonal therapies. Nonetheless, patients with very high indications for failure will benefit from chemotherapy and hormonal therapy sequentially administered.[31] Concurrent administration of hormonal and chemotherapy therapies is also not recommended.[32]

For developing countries, cost is an important factor to be considered in choice of drug as compliance is of importance to attain maximum benefit and prevent drug resistance.

Hormonal therapy: The emergence of third-generation Aromatase Inhibitors

Many breast cancers are oestrogen-dependent and are sensitive to measures to reduce or interfere with oestrogen. In Africans, less than half express hormone receptors.[33]

The options available are:
- Selective Estrogen Receptor Modulators (SERMs);
  - Tamoxifen, Raloxifen,

- Aromatase Inhibitors (AIs) – third generation;
  - ◆ Anastrozole and Letrozole (Non-steroidal),
  - ◆ Exemestane (steroidal),
- Oestrogen Receptor Downregulators (ERDs);
  - ◆ Faslodex,
- Ovarian 'ablation';
  - ◆ Oophorectomy or Radiation.

For many years now tamoxifen, an oestrogen receptor ligand, has had pride of place. It has halved the risk of recurrence and reduced the risk of death by about a quarter in oestrogen receptor -positive patients (EBCTCG 2005).[28] It can however be given for only five years with no added advantage if given longer. Tamoxifen has been available in Ghana and been in use for decades. In the absence of IHC testing for ER/PR status, all breast cancer patients in Ghana were given tamoxifen until recently. Tamoxifen has some undesirable effects which should not be ignored. There are some indications that it may be detrimental if the patient is oestrogen receptor-negative.

In post-menopausal women oestrogen is produced by peripheral conversion from androgens produced by the adrenals, through the activity of aromatase. Aromatase inhibitors (AIs) block aromatase enzyme effectively and thus block oestrogen production. These drugs include anastrozole (arimidex), letrozole (femara) and exemestane (aromasin). Their use is contraindicated in the pre-menopausal setting.[34]

Anastrozole and letrozole have been found to be more effective than tamoxifen in advanced breast cancer.[35] Other trials conducted with multiple arms comparing tamoxifen to third-generation AIs are:

- Upfront trials (Giving one adjuvant drug treatment);
  - ◆ Examples: ATAC, BIG 1.98, TEAM,
- Extended adjuvant trials (Giving AI after completing five years of tamoxifen);
  - ◆ Examples are MA-17, NSABP B33,
- Sequential trials (Giving 2-3 years tamoxifen, then switching to AIs, and vice versa);
  - ◆ Examples are ARNO, ABCSG, IES, BIG 1.98.

These trials have led to the following conclusions in post menopausal women:
1. Upfront anastrozole is superior to tamoxifen;
2. Sequential exemestane or anastrozole after 2-3 years is superior to continued tamoxifen;
3. Extended adjuvant therapy with letrozole after 5 years of tamoxifen further reduces recurrence and improves survival (node +).

All AIs have at least as good a toxicity profile as tamoxifen. There is an increased risk of osteoporosis that appears low and manageable. AIs have a significantly lower association with endometrial cancers and cause less vaginal discharge/bleeding.

These third generation aromatase inhibitors are now the first choice in postmenopausal women with ER+ cancers. The drugs and assessment of bone density and effect of treatment are now available in Accra, Ghana.

Biologic therapy: Trastuzumab

About 20 percent of Africans with breast cancer will express the HER2 gene, localized to chromosome 17q. Amplification of HER2 gene will lead to overexpression of the human epidermal growth factor receptor 2 (HER2), a persistent, independent, negative prognostic factor for breast cancer.[36] Signaling from HER2 receptor will lead to:
• Increased cell proliferation,
• Increased cell migration,
• Resistance to apoptosis,

Trastuzumab (Herceptin®) is a humanized monoclonal antibody, the first targeted therapy for HER2-positive breast cancer. It has doubled the disease free interval and overall survival of patients expressing this gene (3+ or FISH-confirmed 2+).[37] Herceptin targets the transmembrane HER2 receptor to provide clinical benefit, working through cytotoxic and cytostatic mechanisms of action:
• Cytotoxic,
  ♦ Facilitation of immune function by mediating ADCC,
  ♦ Apoptosis,
  ♦ Potentiation of chemotherapy effects,

- Cytostatic,
  ♦ Inhibition of tumor cell proliferation by receptor endocytosis,
  ♦ Anti-angiogenesis.Although trastuzumab can be given for various durations, strong evidence supports 52-week duration of treatment. It has cardiac complications and needs to be monitored closely.

In Ghana, although Herceptin is available, few patients can afford it. Those who receive it opt for a shorter 9-week duration because of cost.

Radiotherapy

It is the medical use of radiation to cure or palliate mostly cancers. There are a few indications for benign conditions. It forms a vital component of multidisciplinary therapy. In the curative setting it is mostly used as adjuvant therapy and monotherapy in the very locally advanced and palliative setting.

However, the delivery of radiation has seen a lot of technical advancement, from the basic use of the cobalt 60 teletherapy machine, which is readily available and easy to maintain in most developing countries, to the sophisticated cone beam therapy using on line CT scan during therapy and other means. In the absence of all other modalities it is the single most effective treatment modality.

In the curative setting its use is always indicated with breast conservation in early breast cancer as discussed above. Several studies with long term follow up data have shown that total mastectomy is equivalent to lumpectomy and radiation therapy in survival and local recurrence parameters.[38] It reduces breast recurrence by 60 percent and 30 percent respectively for early stage and locally advanced resectable or unresectable disease, and has a survival advantage.[39] Even in the event of complete pathological response after neoadjuvant chemotherapy for advanced breast cancer, the omission of local radiotherapy results in a 30 percent rate of local recurrence.[40] Therefore in the absence of absolute contraindications it is not advisable to withhold radiotherapy to the chest wall for locally advanced breast cancer.

Radiotherapy is very effective in palliating distressing symptoms in the latter stages of the disease when there are metastases to the bone, lung and brain. Most recently the role of chemotherapy at end of life has been challenged, but radiotherapy to sites of metastases may still have a role without reducing quality of life. The role of local radiotherapy to the chest wall/breast in the presence of distant metastases is controversial except when there are local symptoms such as bleeding, pain or ulceration.

Timing of radiotherapy is important to ensure optimum benefit. Ideally radiation should be started between 3 to 6 weeks of surgery or completing chemotherapy cycles.[41] The overall benefit is reduced when radiation is done more than 5 months following surgery or last chemotherapy cycle.

Duration of therapy may be from three to six weeks depending on various factors including technical delivery. Recent studies have proven short and long course treatments to be equivalent for early stage cancers. The total dose delivered depends on overall goal of treatment (i.e. curative versus palliative), anticipated toxicity, margin status, size of original tumour, lymphovascular invasion and age. Typically the radiation field includes the chest wall or intact breast and/ or the supraclavicular area. The supraclavicular area is irradiated when there is more than three axillary lymph nodes positive, nodal status is unknown or when there is recurrence of tumour.[42] New techniques include intraoperative radiotherapy to the tumor bed only or partial breast irradiation for older patients with early breast cancer with low risk of recurrence. A lot of effort is put into reducing the dose to lung, heart and contra-lateral breast during treatment to reduce toxicity including the use of 3 Dimensional CT scan planning and Intensity Modulated Radiation Therapy.

Conclusion

Breast cancer is a heterogeneous disease, making treatment rather complex. There have been many new developments with regard to quality of care, screening, pathology, radiology, surgical treatment, staging, hormonal therapy, chemotherapy, radiotherapy and biological therapy.

Although managing breast cancer in a country like Ghana suffers from resource limitations, there must be a constant aspiration to adopt best practices, based on evidence-based recommendations. It is hoped that as our economies get better, our hospitals will be better equipped to handle breast cancer patients. There must be incremental steps at improving quality of care, research, early diagnosis and survival statistics.

References

1. Parkin, D.M., Bray, F. Ferlay, J. and Pisani P. Global cancer statistics, 2002. CA Cancer J Clin. 2005 Mar-Apr; 55(2):74-108.

2. Guidelines for the management of symptomatic breast disease. The Association of Breast Surgery @ BASO, Royal College of Surgeons of England. EJSO. (2005) 31, S1–S21.

3. http://www.nice.org.uk/nicemedia/live/10887/28763/28763.pdf (accessed October 20, 2013) Improving Outcomes in Breast Cancer. Manual Update. National Institute for Clinical Excellence August 2002

4. Varughese, J. and Richman, S. Cancer care inequity for women in resource poor countries. Rev Obstet Gynaecol 2010; 3(3):122-32.

5. Lewison, G. and Sullivan, R. The impact of cancer research: How publications influence UK Cancer clinical guidelines. Br J Cancer. 2008 June 17; 98(12): 1944-50.

6. Stiller, C.A. Survival in patients with breast cancer: those in clinical trials do better. BMJ 1989;299:1056–9.

7. Natale-Pereira, A., Enard, K.R., Nevarez, L. and Jones, L.A. The role of patient navigators in eliminating health disparities. Cancer. 2011 Aug;117(15 Suppl):3541-50.

8. Barrett, B. and McKenna, P. Communicating benefits and risks of screening for prostate, colon, and breast cancer. Fam Med. 2011 Apr;43(4):248-53.

9. Gotzsche, P. C. and Nielsen, M. Screening for breast cancer with mammography. Cochrane Database Syst Rev. 2006; CD001877.

10. Nelson, H.D., Tyne, K., Naik, A., Bougatsos, C. and Chan, B. K. and Humphrey, L. U.S. Preventive Services Task Force. Screening for breast cancer: an update for the U.S. Preventive Services Task Force. Ann Intern Med. 2009 Nov 17;151(10):727-37, W237-42.

11. Mandelblatt, J.S., Cronin, K. A., Bailey, S. et al. Effects of mammography screening under different screening schedules: model estimates of potential benefits and harms. Ann Intern Med. 2009;151:738-47.

12. Yip, C.H., Smith, R.A., Anderson, B.O., et. al. Breast Health Global Initiative Early Detection Panel. Guideline implementation for breast healthcare in low- and middle-income countries: early detection resource allocation. *Cancer.* 2008 Oct 15;113(8 Suppl):2244-56.

13. www. Komen.org/breast cancer/ general recommendations.html

14. Feig S. Comparison of cost and benefits of breast cancer screening with mammography, ultrasound and MRI.Obstet. Gynaecol Clin North Am 2011 March :38(1)179-96.

15. Berg ,W.A., Blume, J. D. and Cormark, J.B. Combined screening with ultrasound and mammography vrs mammogram alone in women with elevated risk of breast cancer. *JAMA.* 2008 May 299(18);2151-63.

16. www.bccancer.bc.ca Breast cancer pathology reporting checklist.

17. Vant Veer, L. J., Dai, H. and Vandelier, M.J. Gene expression profiling predicts clinical outcome of breast cancer. *Nature.* 2002 Jan 31:415(6871);530-6.

18. Fischer, B. Twenty four year follow-up of a randomized trial comparing total mastectomy, lumpectomy and lumpectomy and radiation for the treatment of invasive breast cancer. *N Eng J Med.* 2002;347:1233.

19. Straver, M.E., Rutgers, E.J., Rhodenhuis. S. and Lim, C. The relevance of breast cancer subtypes in the outcomes of Neoadjuvant chemotherapy. Ann Surg Oncol. 2010 Sep; 17 (9): 2411–8.

20. Moy, B. Localized breast cancer. In *Harrison's manual of Oncology.* Chapter 59 pg 521. (Eds). Chabner, B.A., Lynch, T.J., Congo, D.L., McGraw Hill. ISBN 978-0-07-141189-9.

21. Freeman, G., Fowble. B., Hanlon, N. and Fan, D. Patients with early stage invasive cancer with close or positive margins treated with conservation surgery and radiation have an increased risk of breast cancer recurrence that is delayed by adjuvant systemic therapy. *Int J Radiation Oncol Biol Phys.* 1999 July 15; 44 (5)1005-15.

22. Asgeirsson, K.S., Rasheed, T., McCauley, S. J. and Macmillan, R.D. Oncological and cosmetic outcomes of oncoplastic breast conserving surgery *Eur J Surg Oncol* 2005 Oct ;31(8):817-23.

23. Motwani, S.B., Strome, A. and McNeese, M.D. Breast cancer, In *Practical Clinical Applications;Technical basis of Radiation therapy.*Ed Seymour H, Lewit 4th edition , chapter 19 pg 487. Springer ISBN 973-3540-35665-3.

24. Takei, H., Kurosonmi, M. and Yoshida, T. Current trends of sentinel node biopsy for breast cancer - a surgeons perspective.Breast cancer 2007:14(4);362-70.

25. Giuliano, A.E., McCall, L., Beitsch, P., Whitworth, P.W., Blumencranz, P., Leitch. A.M., Saha. S., Hunt, K.K., Morrow, M. and Ballman, K. Locoregional recurrence after sentinel lymph node dissection with or without axillary dissection in patients with sentinel lymph node metastases: the American College of Surgeons Oncology Group Z0011 randomized trial. *Ann Surg.* 2010 Sep;252(3):426-32.

26. Ohene-Yeboah, M. and Adjei, E. Breast cancer in Kumasi, Ghana. *Ghana Med J.* 2012 Mar; 46(1):8-13.

27. Haydaroglu, A., Bolukbari, Y., Demirci, S., Sassolak, M.E. and Ozsaran Z. The prognostic impact of percentage of involved axillary lymph nodes for breast cancer patients treated with radiotherapy. *J Clin Oncol.* 26: 2008(May 20 suppl abst 582).

28. Early Breast Cancer Trialists Collaborative Group (EBCTCG). Effects of chemotherapy and hormonal therapy for early breast cancer on recurrence and 15-year survival: an overview of the randomised trials. *Lancet.* 2005 May 14-20; 365(9472)1687-717.

29. Parikh, P, M., Gupta, S., Parikh, B., Smrut,i B.K., Issrani, J. and Topiwala, S. et al. Management of primary and metastatic triple negative breast cancer: Perceptions of oncologists from India. *Indian J Cancer.* 2011;48:158-64.

30. Brian, R. et al. Cardiac Toxicity in Breast Cancer Survivors: Review of Potential Cardiac Problems. *Clin Cancer Res* January 1, 2008 14:14-24.

31. International Breast Cancer Study Group: Colleoni M, Gelber S, Goldhirsch A, Aebi S, Castiglione-Gertsch M, Price KN, Coates AS, Gelber RD. Tamoxifen After Adjuvant Chemotherapy for Premenopausal Women With Lymph Node-Positive Breast Cancer: *J Clin Oncol.* Mar 20, 2006:1332-1341.

32. Albain, K.S. et tal. Breast Cancer Intergroup of North America. Adjuvant chemotherapy and timing of tamoxifen in postmenopausal patients with endocrine-responsive, node-positive breast cancer: a phase 3, open-label, randomised controlled trial. Lancet. 2009 Dec 19;374(9707):2055-63.

33. Yarney, J., Vanderpuye, V., and Clegg-Lamptey, J. N. Hormone receptor and HER-2 expression in breast cancers among Sub-Saharan African women. *Breast J.* 2008 Oct; 14(5): 510–511.

34. Pinto, M.A., Ballesteros. G.A., Izarzugaza, P.Y., Manso, S.L., Lopez-Tarruella, C.S. et al. Adjuvant hormonal therapy in perimenopausal patients. *Adv Ther.*2011 Sept 28 suppl 6:39-49.

35. Dowsett, M., Cuzick, J., Ingle, J., Coates. A., Forbes, J et al. Meta-Analysis of Breast Cancer Outcomes in Adjuvant Trials of Aromatase Inhibitors Versus Tamoxifen. *J Clin Oncol.* 2010 Jan 20;28(3):509-18.

36. Slamon, D.J. et. al. Human breast cancer: correlation of relapse and survival with amplification of the HER-2/neu oncogene. *Science.* 1987 Jan 9;235(4785):177-82.

37. Hudis, C.A. Trastuzumab - Mechanism of Action and use in clinical practice. *N Eng J* Med2007; 357:39-51.

38. Johansen, H., Kaae. S., Jensen. M.B. and Mouridsen. H,T. Extended radical mastectomy versus simple mastectomy followed by radiotherapy in primary breast cancer. A fifty-year follow-up to the Copenhagen Breast Cancer randomised study. *Acta Oncol.* 2008;47(4):633-8.

39. Clarke, M., Collins, R., Darby, S. et al. Early Breast Cancer Trialists' Collaborative Group (EBCTCG). Effects of radiotherapy and of differences in the extent of surgery for early breast cancer on local recurrence and 15-year survival: an overview of the randomised trials.*Lancet.* 2005 Dec 17; 366 (9503):2087-106.

40. McGuire, S.E., Gonzalez-Angulo, A.M. et al. Postmastectomy Radiation Improves the Outcome of Patients With Locally Advanced Breast Cancer Who Achieve a Pathologic Complete Response to Neoadjuvant Chemotherapy. *Int J Rad Oncol Biol Phy.* July 2007; 68 (4): 1004-9.

41. Punglia, R. S., Saito. A.M., Neville, B.A., Earle, C.C. and Weeks, J. C.et al. Impact of interval from breast conserving surgery to radiotherapy on local recurrence in older women with breast cancer: retrospective cohort analysis. *BMJ.* 2010 Mar 2;340:c845.

42. Yu, J.I., Park, W., Huh, S. J., Choi, D. H., Lim, Y. H. et al. Determining Which Patients Require Irradiation of the Supraclavicular Nodal Area After Surgery for N1 Breast Cancer. *Int J Rad Oncol Biol Phy.* November 2010 (Vol. 78, Issue 4, Pages 1135-41.

Chapter 4
Benign and Premalignant Breast Disease
F. Dedey

Introduction

Breast disease is one of the most common conditions presenting at outpatient clinics worldwide [1] and this also pertains in Ghana.[2, 3, 4] Most of these (72 - 93 percent) are benign.[1, 2, 3, 5, 6] Although females are more commonly affected,[1, 4, 6] some males are also seen with benign breast disease.[6]

Benign breast diseases are now regarded as 'Aberrations of Normal Development and Involution' (ANDI), reflecting the wide spectrum of disorders and diseases which it encompasses. It includes benign diseases without any risk of malignancy (non proliferative breast disease), and those with malignant potential (proliferative breast disease). Non proliferative diseases include common conditions such as fibrocystic changes, cysts, duct ectasia and mastitis. Others are mild hyperplasia, squamous metaplasia, apocrine metaplasia and adenosis. Proliferative diseases include fibroadenoma, moderate/florid hyperplasia, microglandular adenosis, sclerosing adenosis , papilloma (fibrovascular core), atypical ductal hyperplasia and atypical lobular hyperplasia.[7]

One of the aims in the management of these diseases is to identify those with a risk of malignancy and manage them appropriately so as to significantly reduce the incidence and mortality of Breast Cancer.

Assessment

Breast disease is usually assessed with the triple assessment. This includes :

- clinical assessment involving the history and physical examination,

- radiological assessment involving ultrasound and mammogram usually,
- biopsy.

Clinical Assessment

In assessing the patient clinically, certain factors related to the patient may serve as pointers to benign disease. Some of these factors include :

Age - younger patients tend to have benign disease [2,6]

Sex – breast disease is commoner in females and tends to be more often benign, but males may also have benign breast disease commonly gynaecomastia.

Duration – patients with a long history usually have benign disease

Pregnancy or lactation may predispose to certain benign conditions commonly mastitis or breast abscesses.

Menopausal status – benign conditions are more common in premenopausal women.

The symptoms the patient presents with, also helps one to determine which type of breast disease the patient has.

Breast pain, one of the most common symptoms of breast disease[3,4] may be diffuse or specific. It may also be cyclical or not. Majority of patients presenting with pain have benign disease.[4,8] Another common symptom of benign breast disease, breast lumps,[3,4] may be discrete or generalized. Changes in the size of the lump may occur over time. They tend to be more common in the upper outer quadrant of the breast. Nipple discharge is also a common symptom.[3,4] It may be milky or a non milky discharge (clear/ green/ brown/ bloody/ purulent). The discharge may either be unilateral or bilateral, and from solitary or multiple ducts. It occurs more commonly in women with benign breast disease such as fibrocystic changes, intraduct papilloma, duct ectasia, galactorrhea and infection as compared to women with cancer. In the case of the latter the discharge is often bloody. Pathologic nipple discharge is usually spontaneous, persistent and from a single duct or bloody. [9]

In a study of the profile of breast diseases in a self referral clinic in Ghana involving 748 patients, the three most common symptoms at presentation were breast pain, lumps and nipple discharge.[3]

Some of the other symptoms patients may present with include nipple retraction which may be unilateral or bilateral, and tends to be longstanding in benign breast disease, but could also be of recent onset in some conditions. Skin changes such as redness, rashes, ulcers or swelling may also be present. Tenderness, differential warmth and axillary lymphadenopathy may be detected. Other associated symptoms may be fever, malaise, anorexia, vomiting, night sweats and weight loss.

Examination should pay particular attention to the characteristics of any lumps present such as the edges which are usually well defined, the consistency which is often soft or firm, the mobility which is freely mobile without any attachments to surrounding structures and skin and nipple changes and axillary lymph node enlargement.

Radiological Assessment

This involves the use of various radiological techniques to image the breast. The modalities most often employed include:

Ultrasound

This may detect solid or cystic masses and the cystic ones could be either simple or complex.

Benign features include a wider than tall mass, thin echogenic capsule, intense & uniform hyperechogenecity, macro lobulations and smooth margins.

Mammogram

This uses low dose radiation to examine the breasts and may be either for diagnostic or screening purposes.

A universal reporting system, the BIRADS (Breast Imaging Reporting And Data System) is used to classify the abnormality, with increasing likelihood of being benign if the score is low. The scores range from 0 (indeterminate, requiring further studies), through to 6 (an already diagnosed malignancy).

Malignant features include micro calcifications (irregular, clustered, branching), spiculated or irregular masses, skin/nipple changes, axillary node abnormalities, asymmetries and architectural distortions.

Biopsy

Various techniques are available and the most appropriate should be chosen in each situation. It is of utmost importance to be certain of the diagnosis of a benign lesion before treatment is commenced. Malignant lesions which are mistakenly managed as benign ones from the onset complicate the management plan, and may result in worse outcomes. The modalities include :

Fine needle aspiration cytology which uses a small gauge needle to aspirate cells from the area of the abnormality for cytological examination.

Core biopsy which uses a larger bore needle to cut a core of tissue for histological examination.

Excision biopsy which involves surgical removal of the entire area of the abnormality for histological examination. In benign conditions, it serves both to confirm the diagnosis and treat.

Incision biopsy which involves the surgical removal of a portion of the abnormality for histological examination. This is indicated in suspicious ulcers, or where paget's disease or inflammatory breast carcinoma is suspected.

Treatment Options include :
Observation,
Medications,
Aspiration,
Drainage,
Excision,
Mastectomy (rarely).

Screening

This is the process of testing an otherwise healthy woman for breast cancer in an attempt to achieve an earlier diagnosis and hence a better outcome. It therefore involves actively looking for a cancer in women who have no features to suggest the presence of the disease.

Currently no national screening program exits in Ghana.

Modalities for screening include:
• Self breast examination (monthly from 20 years) or self breast awareness;

- Clinical breast examination (3 yearly from 20 – 39 yrs, then annually from 40 yrs, or biannually from 25yrs in high risk patients);
- Mammogram (annually from 40 yrs but earlier for high risk patients) + ultrasound (which reduces the non detectable malignancies from 10-15 percent to 3 percent[7]).

Additionally, Magnetic Resonance Imaging (MRI) can be undertaken annually for high risk women. High risk patients are identified by having had previous significant radiation to the chest, genetic mutations, Lobular Carcinoma In situ (LCIS) and by the use of risk models such as the Gail and Claus risk models[10].

Specific Disorders

Some of the more common specific disorders will be discussed.

Fibrocystic Changes

This is also known as fibroadenosis, mammary dysplasia, cystic mastopathy, chronic cystic disease etc. It is one of the two most common benign breast diseases in females [2] affecting up to 50 percent of premenopausal women usually between 20 – 50 years old. [11]

Common symptoms include cyclical bilateral breast pain, engorgement, fluctuating lumps and nipple discharge especially during the premenstrual phase and relieved with the onset of the menses. Examination reveals general nodularity/lumpiness with tenderness.

Imaging and biopsy may be indicated to rule out malignancy if suspicious.

Treatment options include:

- Reassurance,
- Supportive bra,
- Topical NSAIDS,
- Evening primrose oil,
- Danazol, Bromocriptin or Tamoxifen if very severe and
- Decreased intake of methylxanthines. This is controversial but has been found to be beneficial in some studies.

Fibroadenoma

This is the other of the two most common benign breast diseases, occurring in the 2nd and 3rd decades. It usually grows slowly, about 30 percent will disappear while approximately 10 percent become smaller. The rest either remain the same in size or increase.About 15 percent of the lumps are multiple and 20 percent recur after excision [12]. Giant fibroadenoma is more than 5cm in diameter.[13]

Features include firm, rubbery, well defined, solid and freely mobile lumps (also referred to as the breast mouse). It is neither painful, nor tender and does not fluctuate in size.

Treatment options include excision biopsy commonly or conservative management for small lumps in patients less than 35 years and with the diagnosis confirmed by clinical, imaging and biopsy. Regular follow up is necessary if the conservative option is chosen.

Phyllodes Tumour

It is also referred to as cystosarcoma phyllodes or brodie's tumor. It is commoner in the 5th decade. It is rapidly growing and maybe benign (60 percent), borderline (15 percent) or malignant-(1 in 4).[12] Only few of the malignant lesions metastasize to lungs, liver and bones. It presents as a large well defined lump, with dilated veins on the skin, without enlarged axillary lymph nodes. Treatment is to excise widely. Mastectomy may be indicated if the margins are positive, or histology is borderline/ malignant. Recurrence is common even for benign tumors, hence the need for wide excision.

Cysts

These usually occur in women more than 35 years old, but may occur in older women using exogenous hormones. They are well defined painless and mobile lumps. Treatment is by aspiration. If bloody, a residual mass occurs, or there is recurrence of the cyst, aspirate is sent for cytology. Excision biopsy may be required for complex cysts, a residual mass or recurrent cyst after aspiration. Intracyst carcinomas occur very rarely in about 0.1 percent of cases.[13]

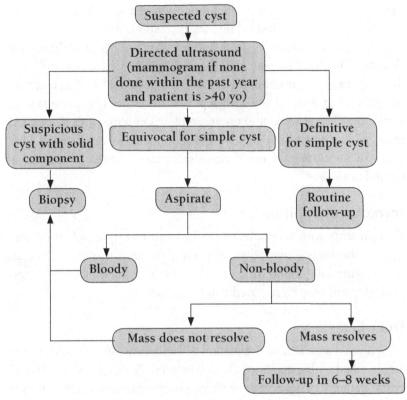

Figure 4.1: Algorithm for the management of suspected cysts [7]

Galactocele

This is a milk containing cyst, with inspissated milk accumulated in the ducts, which is well circumscribed and mobile. It usually occurs after cessation of lactation or with reduction in frequency of feeding. Needle aspiration is usually done or surgery, if it cannot be aspirated or is infected.

Mastitis /Breast Abscess

This usually occurs in lactating and pregnant women (malignancy or immunocompromise should be excluded if the patient is not in the peripartum period). Non lactational mastitis and abscesses may also be associated with duct ectasia and smoking. Staphylococci or streptococci are the usual offending organisms, but rarely other bacteria, fungi or acid fast bacilli may be responsible.

Antibiotic treatment is given and incision and drainage done for abscess collections. Biopsy of abscess wall is indicated in patients more than 40 years old, or not in the peripartum period. Duct excision may be required in duct ectasia with repeated infection. It is important to remember that chronic abscess resemble carcinoma with ill defined mass, peau d'orange and axillary lymph nodes. Hence the need once again to be certain of the diagnosis before definitive treatment is carried out.

Intraductal Papilloma

This presents with spontaneous intermittent bloody nipple discharge from a unilateral solitary duct. It usually occurs beneath the areolar. It is commonly found in perimenopausal women. Cytology and mammogram may be required before excision.

Duct Ectasia

It involves distension and dilatation of lactiferous sinuses beneath the areola, filled with inspissated cheesy material. Peak age is from 40 – 50 years. Patients present with recurrent breast pain/discomfort, nipple discharge, nipple retraction, retroareolar mass, mamillary fistula with or without an abscess and enlarged axillary lymph nodes. It may also resemble a carcinoma. Treatment is by microdocectomy or hadfields operation (cone excision of the ducts).

Fat Necrosis

History of trauma is usually not obtained although it is said to be caused by trauma. It presents with a painless, hard, irregular mass, which may be attached to skin, with ill defined edges. It is also a differential for carcinoma. A core biopsy to confirm the diagnosis may be required. An excision biopsy may also be done.

Tietze's Syndrome

This involves Inflammation of the costochondrial junctions usually involving the 2^{nd}one. There is localized tenderness on palpation. Reassurance and pain relief is given.

Mondor's Disease

Thrombophlebitis of the superficial breast veins namely, lateral thoracic, thoracoepigastric and superficial epigastrics. Examination reveals a palpable tender cord going into the axilla. Approximately 25 percent of cases may have an associated malignancy, so thorough investigations must be carried out. Anti inflammatory agents, warm compress, supportive bra and restriction of movement are helpful.

Gynaecomastia

The most common breast disease in men [2] is an enlarged breast which may be unilateral or bilateral. It usually occurs either in the neonatal, adolescent or senescent periods due to excess circulating estrogens over testosterone in these periods of male development. This may result from excess estrogen or deficient androgen states eg tumors, systemic diseases, congenital abnormalities, medications and testicular failure. The above possible causes must be excluded as well as breast malignancy. Treatment of any underlying cause must be undertaken. Reassurance only, may suffice or mastectomy may be indicated usually for cosmetic reasons.

Other common superficial benign disorders occurring elsewhere in the body may also be present in the breast. These include:
- Lipoma which is a soft, lobulated, well defined mass.
- Sebacous cyst which is a well defined mass attached to skin with a punctum.
- Eczema which is usually bilateral and occurs during lactation. There is associated pruritus and vesicles. The nipple is intact with no breast lumps as compared to paget's disease which is malignant.

- Accessory breasts which presents as a mass usually in the axilla that enlarges in pregnancy. Excision is indicated for cosmetic reasons usually.

Premalignant Disorders

All of these disorders possess some malignant properties, but lack the ability to invade and metastasize which is characteristic of malignant disease.[14, 15] These conditions are not frequently diagnosed in our Subregion, partly due to lack of national screening programs. [11]

They include:

Atypical ductal hyperplasia (ADH),

Atypical lobular hyperplasia (ALH),

Ductal carcinoma in situ (DCIS),

Lobular carcinoma in situ (LCIS),

Atypical Ductal / Lobular Hyperplasia (ADH/ALH).

This is proliferative breast disease with 4 - 5 X increased risk of breast cancer for atypical ductal hyperplasia and 5.8 X increased risk for atypical lobular hyperplasia. This risk is doubled if a 1st degree relative has breast cancer. [14] It may be difficult to differentiate from in situ disease. Also, up to 20 percent of cases will have carcinoma and therefore excision of the lesion is required. [7]

Ductal Carcinoma In Situ (DCIS)

DCIS has all the cellular features of carcinoma but without invasion. It has increased from 5 percent to ~20 percent of cancer cases.[7] Untreated, 60 – 100 percent of DCIS will progress to invasive cancer, with 10 percent mortality at 10 yrs. [14] Majority, (90 percent) of cases are diagnosed by mammogram with only 10 percent presenting with palpable masses.[16] For those diagnosed by mammogram, 75 percent have clustered calcifications, 10 percent have mammographic densities while 15 percent show both.[13] To confirm the diagnosis histologically, needle biopsy usually by wire localisation is necessary. The specimen is radiographed after biopsy, to ensure the abnormality has been sampled. It must be noted that up to 20 percent of DCIS diagnosed by needle biopsy have invasive carcinoma on excision.[17] Without invasion however, the risk of metastasis is negligible.

In treatment of DCIS, several factors [16, 17, 18] should be considered to determine the type of treatment to give. The histologic type such as the comedo type is likely to present as a palpable mass and be of high grade and hence be invasive, while the micropapillary type is often multicentric. These may therefore require more aggressive treatment as compared to the others such as the cribiform, solid and papillary types. The grade, extent of the lesion, estrogen receptor status, microinvasion and patients' age and preference also guide the clinician as to what treatment options to use.

A multidisciplinary team comprising of a surgeon, pathologist, oncologist, radiologist and nurses is necessary for effective treatment [17].

Predictors of recurrence include [16, 17] young age, positive family history, positive margins (29 percent recurrence as against 7 percent with negative margins), histologic subtype (eg comedo necrosis), Van Nuys Prognostic Index (takes into account the size, margin and histology) and estrogen receptor & HER 2 status.

Treatment Options include:

1.   Breast Conservation only.

The Van Nuys criteria was developed to identify patients who would benefit from breast conservation alone without radiotherapy, using grade, size, age and margin width. Studies have however not been reproduced.

2.   Breast Conservation with Radiotherapy (RT)

Radiotherapy decreases recurrence from 16.4 percent to 7 percent with 8 year follow up and invasive cancer from 8 percent to 2 percent - (NSABP B-17). Radiotherapy benefits have also been shown by the European Organization for Research and Treatment of Cancer - EORTC 10853 and SWEDICS trials. RT should be started 2 – 4 weeks post operatively.[13]

19% of patients who have conservation recur with half of them as invasive disease. Treatment is to excise and radiate if no prior RT was given. If RT was given and recurrence is non invasive, total mastectomy is indicated, but if invasive disease occurs, then axillary surgery should be done together with the mastectomy.[16]

3. Simple Mastectomy

This has a 1 percent local recurrence.[7] Indications include [13, 17] diffuse calcifications, positive margins on conservation, likelihood of poor cosmetic result, patient preference and contraindications to radiotherapy.

4. Axillary Lymph Node Dissection (ALND)

This is contraindicated as only <5 percent [17] have positive nodes. These patients with positive nodes are usually found to have invasive disease. Invasion is more likely with extensive high grade DCIS or a palpable mass. [16, 17]

5. Sentinel Lymph Node Dissection (SLND)

This is indicated when mastectomy is carried out, microinvasion is detected and / or extensive calcification is present, especially with a high grade lesion and a palpable mass.

6. Hormonal Therapy (HT)

This prevents new primaries and improves local control.

Tamoxifen is indicated for ER positives with conservation (NSABP – 24 showed a 43 percent decrease in invasive Breast Cancer and 31 percent decrease in non invasive events. Also 30 percent decrease in ipsilateral and 52 percent decrease in contralateral events.)

Patients at highest risk of recurrence, that is those with positive margins, comedo necrosis, a mass and those less than 50 years benefit more from hormonal treatment if indicated. However, deep vein thrombosis and endometrial cancer, the side effects of hormonal treatment (tamoxifen) should be considered. Hence, the benefits should be weighed against the risks of treatment before its commencement.

Follow up is done 6 monthly for 5-8 years, then annually with an annual mammogram. [16, 17]

7. Lobular carcinoma in situ (LCIS)

LCIS usually occurs in premenopausal women (90 percent) between 40 and 50 years, as an incidental finding (it has no clinical nor radiological features). 50 percent are multifocal and 30 percent are bilateral.[7, 14] There is an 8-10X risk of breast cancer, usually occurring as ductal carcinoma. This carcinoma may occur in either breast hence LCIS is considered to be a risk factor for carcinoma and not strictly a premalignant condition.[7] A 30 – 35 percent cumulative risk of developing breast cancer exists in patients with LCIS. Untreated, 15 percent develop ipsilateral cancer and 9 percent contralateral disease.[19]

Treatment options for LCIS include :[7]

1. Close Observation, which enables early detection of carcinoma Chemoprophylaxis with tamoxifen or raloxifen which decreases the risk by 50 - 70 percent. The side effect profile of raloxifene is better than that of estrogen. (NSABP P1 , P2) and

2. Bilateral Prophylactic Mastectomy which markedly reduces the risk of carcinoma but does not completely eliminate it.

References

1. Memon, A., Parveen S., Sangrasi, A.K., Malik Aziz, A.,Laghari Altaf, K., Talpur, H., Ali, Q.G. Changing Pattern of Benign Breast Lumps in Young Females. *American-Eurasian Journal of Scientific Research* . 2007; 2 (1): 52-56.

2. Asumanu, E., Vowotor, R., and Naeder, S. B. Pattern of Breast Disease in Ghana. *Ghana Medical Journal.* December 2000; 34(4): 206 - 209

3. Clegg –Lamptey J. N. A., Aduful, H. K., Yarney, J. et al. Profile of breast diseases at a self-referral clinic in Ghana. *West African Journal of Medicine.* March 2009; 28(2) : 114-7.

4. Ohene-Yeboah, M. and Amaning, E. P. Spectrum of complaints presented at a specialist breast clinic in Kumasi, Ghana. *Ghana Medical Journal,* September 2008; 42(3): 110–113.

5. Ohene-Yeboah, M. O. K. An audit of excised breast lumps in Ghanaian women. *West African Journal of Medicine.* July - September 2005; 24 (3) : 252 - 255.

6. Olu-Eddo, A. N. and Ugiagbe, E. E. Benign breast lesions in an African population: A 25-year histopathological review of 1864 cases. *Nigerian Medical Journal.* 2011;52 (4):211-6.

7. Lewis .J. and Borgen, P. Breast Disease in Women's Health. In : Bope and Kellerman: *Conn's Current Therapy.* 1st ed. Saunders 2012, 985 - 993.

8. Clegg – Lamptey, J. N. A., Edusa C., Ohene-Nti, N. and Tagoe, J. A. Breast Cancer Risk in Patients with Breast Pain in Accra, Ghana. *East African Medical Journal.* May 2007; 84(5): 215 - 218.

9. Santen, R. J. and Mansel, R. Benign Breast Disorders. *New England Journal of Medicine.* July 2005; 353 (3):275-285.

10. Pichert, G., Bolliger, B., Buser, K and Pagani, O. Evidence-based management options for women at increased breast/ovarian cancer risk. *Annals of Oncology.* 2003; 14 (1): 9–19.

11. Goehring, C. Morabia A. Epidemiology of Benign Breast Disease, with Special Attention to Histologic Types. Epidemiologic Reviews by *The Johns Hopkins University School of Hygiene and Public Health.* 1997 ; 19(2) : 310 - 327.

12. Katz, V. L. and Dotter,s D. Breast Diseases. In Lentz, Lobo, Gershenson and Katz: *Comprehensive Gynecology.* 6th ed.; Mosby 2012, 301 - 334

13. Iglehar,t J. D. and Smith, B. L. Diseases of the Breast. In : Townsend, Beauchamp, Evers and Mattox (eds) : *Sabiston Textbook of Surgery, The Biological Basis of Modern Surgical Practice.* 18th ed. Saunders 2007.

14. Vecchione L. Premalignant Disease : The Breast. *Journal of Insurance Medicine.* 1999; 31:21-24.

15. Allred, D. C., Mohsin, S.O., Fuqua, S. A. Histological and Biological Evolution of Human Premalignant Breast Disease. Endocrine - Related Cancer. 2001; (8) 47 – 61.

16. Winchester D. P, Jeske J. M, Goldschmidt R. A. The diagnosis and management of ductal carcinoma in-situ of the breast. May/June 2000; 50 (3): 184 – 200.

17. Morrow, M., Strom, E. A., Bassett, L. W., Dershaw, D. D., Fowble. B. Harris, J. R., O'Malley, .F, Schnitt, S.. J., Singletary, S.. E. and Winchester, D. P. Standard for management of Ductal Carcinoma In-Situ of the breast. *A Cancer Journal for Clinicians.* Sept/Oct 2002; 52 (5): 256 – 276.

18. Donohue, J. H. Management of ductal carcinoma in situ .*Journal of Breast Health,* 2006; 2(1) : 52 -53.

19. Shin, S. J, Rosen P. P. Excisional biopsy should be performed if LCIS is seen on Needle Core Biopsy. *Archives of pathology and Laboratory Medicine.* June 2002;126 (6) : 697 - 701.

Chapter 5
Acute Appendicitis
S.B. Naaeder, J.N. Clegg-Lamptey and J.C.B. Dakubo

Introduction

In 1886 Reginald H. Fitz first described appendicitis in his presentation titled "Perforating inflammation of the vermiform appendix with special reference to its early diagnosis and treatment" to the first meeting of the Association of American Physicians in Washington DC[1]. He coined the term appendicitis to distinguish it from other inflammatory conditions in the region of the caecum such as typhilitis and perityphilitis. This was followed by Charles McBurney's description of his classical sign in the diagnosis of acute appendicitis in 1889[2]. Appendicitis is now the most common intra-abdominal emergency surgical condition worldwide. It has been postulated that acute appendicitis is the first serious disease to emerge following dietary modification with the adoption of fibre-depleted diets. In 1920 Rendle Short propounded the hypothesis that the rise in the incidence of acute appendicitis in western populations was primarily due to the substitution of high-residue diets with refined low-fibre diets.[3] This concept was popularized by Dennis Burkitt[4] who reviewed all the available epidemiological and experimental evidence and concluded that undue refining of dietary carbohydrate was the most important causative factor of acute appendicitis, diverticular disease and large bowel cancer. He noted the rarity of these large bowel diseases in African populations who consumed diets high in fibre and the high incidence of these diseases in populations living on low fibre diets.[4] The incidence of acute appendicitis is rising in Africa and this has been attributed to socio-economic advancement with its accompanying life-style changes and adoption of low-residue diets. However, current evidence suggests that low-residue diet may not be the important aetiological factor in acute appendicitis as has been postulated. This is because, in Africa, patients with acute appendicitis consume traditional high -residue diets and urbanization has been shown to have no effect on the dietary fibre intake and bowel function of Africans[5].

Incidence

There is considerable variation in the incidence of appendicitis all over the world. The disease is common in western nations but much less so in developing countries, however, this is changing. Recent reports suggest that the incidence of acute appendicitis is declining in the developed world. The reason for this decline is not clear but it has been suggested that this may be related to an increase in dietary fibre intake in these populations[6]. Between 1989 and 2000 the age-standardized hospital admission rates for acute appendicitis in England was noted to have decreased by 12.5 per cent in males and 18.8 percent in females[7]. In the USA the incidence of appendicitis decreased by 14.6 per cent between 1970 and 1984.[6] All reports on acute appendicitis were unanimous that acute appendicitis was rare in Africa six to seven decades ago.[8,9] This is no longer the situation as the incidence of the disease has been increasing progressively ever since. Adekunle O.O et al. reported a progressive increase in the annual incidence of acute appendicitis in Nigeria between 1973 and 1983[10]. Similar trends have been reported in both rural and urban communities in Ghana[11-15] and other parts of Africa.[16-17] Acute appendicitis was uncommon in Ghana in the 1940s; by 1966 the annual incidence was 2.2 per 10,000 population.[12] This rose to 2.63 per 10,000 population by 1971[13] and currently the reported annual incidence of acute appendicitis is 3.18 per 10,000 population.[14] This is still lower than the annual incidence rate of 11 per 10,000 population reported in the USA with an even higher rate (25 per 10,000 population) in the young (10-19 years).[6] Acute appendicitis is now the leading cause of the acute abdomen in Africa including the West African sub-region[18-21].

Aetiology of acute appendicitis

The cause of appendicitis has been attributed to a number of factors. Diets low in residue have been blamed[4] but studies in Ghana have disputed this notion.[5,22] These studies noted that urbanization had no effect on the dietary habits of Ghanaians and that dietary fibre intake was high in patients with acute appendicitis. Gelfand found that patients admitted with acute appendicitis in Africa followed a traditional diet.[23] Appendicular luminal obstruction is thought to initiate the inflammatory changes associated with acute appendicitis. The obstruction is by a faecolith in the majority of cases but it may be due to lymphoid hyperplasia following viral infections, respiratory tract infections or gastroenteritis especially in children and young adults. Obstruction may also be due to adhesions with kinking of the appendix, stricture within its lumen and rarely due to parasites, foreign bodies or carcinoid tumour. Appendicitis is most common in the second and third decades[5,14,24] and less so in those under 2 years and above 40 years. Males are its commonest victims, being up to two times more as common in males than in females.[14,15,24]

Clinical features

The diagnosis of acute appendicitis is largely clinical. The symptomatology of acute appendicitis has not changed over the years. The presenting features are typical and are essentially the same everywhere in the world. Pain is the main and leading symptom in all cases and is typically periumbilical and colicky due to obstruction of the lumen of the appendix or a dull ache from catarrhal non-obstructive inflammation of the appendix but it may be generalized or even epigastric.[25,26] It then shifts to the right iliac fossa after a variable period. Yet in others it may start in the right iliac fossa and remain there[10,25,26]. It is initially visceral and vague since the appendix is a midgut structure with innervations from the tenth thoracic segment but after migration to the right iliac fossa the pain becomes somatic, constant, sharp and precise. The pain is aggravated by movement and coughing (Dunphy's sign). The description of this classical migration is credited to John Benjamin Murphy[27] but it is noted in only 50 per cent of patients in Western societies.[28] Some reports in Africa found this classical migration to be present in only 37-48 percent of cases.[10,26] In West Africa a previous history of similar attack is not uncommon and has been reported in about a quarter to a third of patients.[10,13,26] The somatic or parietal pain in appendicitis is related to the position of the appendix which has been found to be variable in various reports in Africa and elsewhere.[5,14,29] Thus apart from the right iliac fossa, the somatic pain may be located in the hypogastrium if the appendix is in the pelvic position, lumbar if high retrocaecal and right hypochondrial if subhepatic. In those complicated by generalized peritonitis, the pain involves the entire abdomen.

In Africa, as elsewhere, anorexia is a prominent feature, followed by nausea and vomiting.[10,26,29,30] The latter may be marked if the appendicitis is complicated by generalized peritonitis, otherwise vomiting may be once or twice. Fever is present in a little over half (52 percent) of the cases.[10,30] A slightly lower figure (47 percent) was reported in a more recent study in Ghana.[26] Constipation is variable occurring in about a third to just under 50 percent of patients, whilst diarrhoea is present in some 14-17 percent of cases.[10,13] However, in one study in Ghana the incidence of diarrhoea was as high as 37 percent.[26] In these patients with diarrhoea the inflamed appendix is either in the pelvic or ileal position or there is an associated appendix abscess.[10,13] A pelvic appendix may also cause frequency and dysuria if it lies in contact with the bladder and has been noted in 16.7 percent of patients in Accra[26] but in only 1.4 percent of patients in Nigeria.[24]

In Ghana and West Africa delay in presentation is not uncommon. Some 40 percent of patients now present within 24 hours compared to 17 percent four decades ago.[5,13,26] However there has been no change in the incidence of complicated appendicitis over the years. In 1971 Badoe reported a 43 percent incidence of complicated appendicitis in patients presenting with acute appendicitis in Accra.[13] This incidence rate has remained virtually unchanged as Naaeder et al. in 1998 and 1999 found that 42.8 percent and 41.6 percent of their patients with appendicitis respectively presented with complicated appendicitis.[5,18] This is a sad reflection on the state of our health education system with regards to this common surgical emergency. In Nigeria similar delays in presentation and complicated appendicitis rates are reported.[24,31,32]

The patient may look unwell with the right hip in the flexed position, extension of which worsens the pain (Psoas sign). The temperature is low grade but may be 38°C or more in 44 percent of cases.[26] The tongue is coated and the typical appendicular foetor may be present. Tachycardia is a common feature. Tenderness over the site of the inflamed appendix is the earliest and most important single abdominal sign.[26,33] The location of the tenderness varies with the position of the appendix. In those with a pelvic appendix, tenderness in the right side of the rectum may be elicited on rectal examination. Rebound tenderness and muscle guarding are other clinical signs and usually signify parietal peritoneal irritation. Dunphy's and Rovsing's signs may be elicited. Of the symptoms and signs of acute appendicitis, migration of pain and peritoneal irritation have been found to be the most important diagnostic features and should be considered in all diagnostic assessment of acute appendicitis.[34]

Diagnosis of acute appendicitis in children, the elderly and in late pregnancy may present a formidable challenge and therefore a high index of suspicion is necessary. The disease is uncommon in the very young and peaks in the 10-14 year group.[14,24] Restlessness, anorexia, vomiting, pyrexia, tachycardia, tenderness and guarding are prominent features. Rectal tenderness is a valuable sign. Appendicitis is also uncommon in the aged[13,14,24] in whom the symptoms are atypical and tenderness is less marked. In the third trimester of pregnancy, upward and lateral displacement of the appendix by the gravid uterus may lead to diagnostic difficulties. In all three categories delay in diagnosis is associated with a high incidence of complications.

In all patients, acute appendicitis must be differentiated from other causes of the acute abdomen of which there are many.[18,19] In Africa and elsewhere, the most important differential diagnosis surgeons have to make is that between acute appendicitis and a variety of self-limiting acute abdominal conditions (Non-specific abdominal pain) which do not require prompt surgical intervention.[18,35]

Investigations

The cornerstone in the diagnosis of acute appendicitis has been predominantly clinical and no sophisticated investigations are required in the majority of cases. However ancillary investigations may be required to improve the accuracy of diagnosis and minimize the negative appendicectomy rate which has been reported in some studies to be as high as

15-30 percent. [25,36] In other studies the negative appendicectomy rate was found to be 4-4.5 percent.[5,18]

Laboratory Tests

Reports in western literature put the white cell count levels in acute appendicitis at greater than $10,000/m^3$ in 80-85 percent of cases with a neutrophilia in some 75-80 percent of patients.[37,38] In Ghana and West Africa a white count above $10,000/m^3$ was found in only 44-48 percent of cases with neutrophilia of over 70 percent reported in 73 percent of patients[10,26]. The above reports together with the fact that leucocytosis and neutropilia occur in other intra-abdominal inflammatory conditions mean that white cell count is of low specificity and has low predictive value in the diagnosis of acute appendicitis. C-reactive protein levels are frequently elevated in acute appendicitis and levels above 0.8mg/dl are usual. The finding of leucocytosis, neutrophilia and elevated C-reactive protein levels increases the likelihood of a correct diagnosis of acute appendicitis to 97-100 percent.[28] The drawback in Ghana and West Africa is that C-reactive protein estimation is not done routinely in the evaluation of patients with acute appendicitis. Routine urine examination has been advocated by some as pyuria, haematuria and proteinuria may be present and thus differentiate urinary tract causes of abdominal pain from acute appendicitis. A pregnancy test may be helpful in women in the reproductive age to exclude gynaecological causes of abdominal pain.

Radiological investigations

Radiological support may be necessary in situations in which the diagnosis is uncertain. Ultrasonography and computed tomography of the abdomen have come to replace plain abdominal x-rays and barium enema in the radiological investigation of acute appendicitis. Helical CT scanning, with contrast enhancement, is reported to be superior to ultrasonography in diagnostic accuracy as the latter is operator dependent.[39] However some studies indicate that ultrasonography and computed tomography have not been associated with a reduced negative appendicectomy rate,[40] whereas others have reported a reduction in unnecessary admissions and appendicectomies.[41]

In Ghana and West Africa and indeed, Sub-saharan Africa these radiological investigations are not routinely deployed in the diagnosis of acute appendicitis largely due to resource constraints and cost.

Treatment

The treatment of acute appendicitis is appendicectomy after adequate resuscitation (Figure 1). Antibiotic prophylaxis is exhibited in all patients in order to reduce the incidence of postoperative surgical site infections. Appendicectomy is the commonest emergency surgical operation in both developing and developed countries and is the treatment of choice. It may be done through conventional open surgery or laparoscopically. The latter is increasingly employed in Western nations but in Ghana and most of Africa, laparoscopic surgery is still in its teething stages. The natural history of acute appendicitis includes spontaneous resolution and in a resource-limited setting, antibiotic therapy may be considered for early acute appendicitis with elective appendicectomy later. The latter is recommended because of the high recurrence rates, 24-35 percent associated with conservative management alone.[42-43] In those presenting with an appendix mass the treatment is initially non-operative followed by interval appendicectomy in 6-8 weeks. However, if the patient's condition deteriorates during the period of conservative management, immediate laparotomy is advised. An appendix mass which fails to resolve in two weeks may be ominous and carcinoma of the caecum should be excluded. A small appendix abscess may resolve with antibiotic therapy. Failure to do so and in those with large abscesses percutaneous drainage under ultrasound guidance is done. Where this is unsuccessful, open drainage and appendicectomy, if the appendix can be found, is undertaken. Interval appendicectomy is carried out in cases where the appendix has not been excised. In Ghana and West Africa, the incidence of patients presenting with appendix masses or abscesses has declined from a high of 30 percent in the 1960s [12,13] to between 13 percent and 16 percent in the eighties[10] and nineties[5,18] to 6.4 percent in recent times.[26] This is largely due to a progressive increase in the proportion of patients reporting within 24 hours of onset of symptoms.[5,10,13,26]

The incidence of perforation or gangrene increases with the duration of symptoms, being highest in those presenting after 2 or more days.

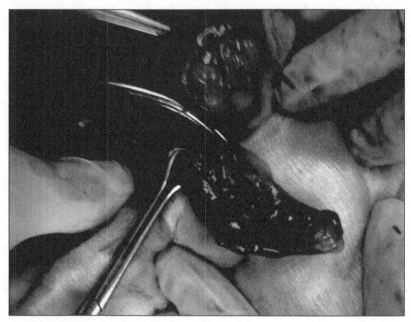

Figure 5.1: Appendicectomy being done for acute appendicitis

Complications

Mortality from appendicectomy is low in West Africa (1-1.3 percent overall) [5,10,14] and is comparable to mortality rates elsewhere.[28] The rates are higher in those with perforation and peritonitis.[13] The causes of death are usually septicaemia and circulatory failure. Wound complication is the most common morbidity following appendicectomy being higher in those with perforation and gangrene. It varies from 8.7 percent to 22 percent in West Africa.[10,14] Other complications include pelvic abscess, fistula and pneumonia.

References

1. Fitz, R. Perforating inflammation of the vermiform appendix with special reference to its early diagnosis and treatment. *Trans. Assoc. Am. Physicians.* 1886; 1: 107-44.

2. McBurney, C. Experiences with early operative interference in cases of diseases of the vermiform appendix. *N.Y. Med. J.* 1889; 50: 676-84.

3. Rendle, S.A. The causation of appendicitis. *Br. J. Surg.* 1920; 8: 171-8.

4. Burkitt, D.P. The aetiology of appendicitis. *Br. J. Surg.* 1971; 58: 695-9.

5. Naaeder, S.B, and Archampong, E.Q.. Acute appendicitis and dietary fibre intake. *West Afr. J. Med.* 1998; 17: 264-7.

6. Adiss, D.G., Shaffer, N., Fowler, B.S. and Tauxe, R.V. The epidemiology of appendicitis and appendectomy in the United States. *Am. J. Epidemiol.* 1990; 132: 910-25.

7. Kang, J.Y., Hoare J., Majeed, A., Williamson, R. C., Maxwell, J.D. Decline in admission rates for acute appendicitis in England. *Br. J. Surg.* 2003; 90: 1586-92.

8. Muller, S. Geographical aspects of appendicitis. *Acta Chirurgica Scand.* 1956; 221: 10-8.

9. Walker, A.P.R., Richardson, B.D., Walker, B.F. and Woolford, A. Appendicitis, fibre intake and bowel behavior in ethnic groups in South Africa. *Postgrad. Med. J.* 1973; 49: 243-9.

10. Adekunle, O.O., and Funmilayo, J. A. Acute appendicitis in Nigeria. *J. R. Coll. Surg. Edin.* 1986; 31: 102-5.

11. Gibney, E.J. Acute appendicitis in rural Ghana: a retrospective study. *Ghana Medical Journal* 1988; 22: 80-4.

12. Badoe, E.A. Acute appendicitis in Accra. *Ghana Medical Journal* 1967; 6: 69-75.

13. Badoe, E.A. Acute appendicitis in Accra, 1967-1969. *Ghana Medical Journal* 1971; 10: 265-69.

14. Clegg-Lamptey, J.N.A, and Naeder, S. B. Appendicitis in Accra: A contemporary appraisal. *Ghana Medical Journal* 2003; 37: 52-6.

15. Ohene-Yeboah, M. and Abantanga, F. A. Incidence of acute appendicitis in Kumasi, *Ghana. West Afr. J. Med.* 2009; 28: 122-25.

16. McConkey, S.J. Case series of acute abdominal surgery in rural Sierra Leone. *World J. Surg.* 2002; 26: 509-13.

17. Awori, M. N, Jani, P. G. Surgical implications of abdominal pain in patients presenting to the Kenyatta National Hospital casualty department with abdominal pain. *E. Afr. Med. J.* 2005; 82: 307-10.

18.   Naaeder S.B, Archampong, E.Q. Clinical spectrum of acute abdominal pain in Accra, Ghana. *West Afr. J. Med.* 1999; 18: 13-16.

19.   Ohene-Yeboah, M. Acute surgical admissions for abdominal pain in adults in Kumasi, Ghana. *ANZ J. Surg.* 2006; 76: 898-903.

20.   Archampong, E.Q. The outcome of peritonitis in an urban medical centre. *Ghana Medical Journal* 1979; 18: 226-9.

21.   Olumide, F., Akande, B., Odugbemi, O. and Adesola, Acute abdomen in Lagos, Nigeria. Changing pattern in an African community. *Ghana Medical Journal* 1980; 19: 98-104.

22.   Opare-Obisaw, C., Fianu, D.A.G. and Awadzi. K. . Changes in family food habits: the role of migration. *J. of Consumer Studies and Home Economics.* 2008; 24: 145-9.

23.   Gelfand, M. The patterns of disease in Africa. *Central Afr. J. Med.* 1971; 17: 69-78.

24.   Edino, S.T., Mohammed, A.Z., Ochicha, O. and Anumah, M. Appendicitis in Kano, Nigeria: A 5-year review of pattern, morbidity and mortality. *Annals of African Medicine.* 2004; 3:38-41.

25.   Ohene-Yeboah, M. and Togbe, B. An audit of appendicitis and appendicectomy in Kumasi, Ghana. *West Afr. J. Med.* 2006; 25: 138-43.

26.   Clegg-Lamptey, J.N.A. Clinical features of acute appendicitis: A two-year study in a Surgical Unit at Korle Bu Teaching Hospital. *Ghana Medical Journal.* 2002; 36: 164-7.

27.   Murphy, J. Two thousand operations for appendicitis, with deductions from his personal experience. *Am. J. Med. Sci.* 1904; 128: 187-211.

28.   Harding, D.M, J.R. Acute appendicitis: Review and update. *Am. Fam. Physician.* 1999; 60: 2027-34.

29.   Fashina, L.B. et al. Acute appendicitis in Lagos: A review of 250 cases. *Niger Postgrad Med J.* 2009; 16: 268-73.

30.   Archampong, E.Q. Peritonitis: Preliminary report 1877 cases. *Ghana Medical Journal.* 1973; 12: 31-41.

31.   Ayoade, B.A., Olawoye, O.A., Salami, B.A. and Banjo, A.A. Acute appendicitis in Olabisi Onabanjo University Teaching Hospital,Sagamu, a three year review. *Niger. J. Clin. Pract.* 2006, 9: 52-6.

32.   Out, A. A. Tropical surgical abdominal emergencies: acute appendicitis. *Trop. Geogr. Med.* 1989; 41: 118-22.

33.   Naaeder, S.B. In: Badoe, E.A., Archampong, E.Q. and da Rocha-Afodu, J.T. (eds.) *Principles and Practice of Surgery Including Pathology in the Tropics.* Accra. Assemblies of God Literature Centre Ltd. 2009: 561-71.

34. Andersson, R.E.B. Meta-analysis of the clinical and laboratory diagnosis of appendicitis. *Br. J. Surg.* 2004; 91: 28-37.
35. Irvin, T.T. Abdominal pain: a surgical audit of 1190 emergency admissions. *Br. J. Surg.* 1989; 76: 1121-25.
36. Malt, R.A. The perforated appendix. *N. Eng. J. Med.* 1986; 315: 1546-7.
37. Sasso, R.D, Hanna, E.A., and Moore, D.L. Leucocytic and neutrophilic counts in acute appendicitis. *Am. J. Surg.* 1970; 120: 563-6.
38. Elangovan, S. Clinical and laboratory findings in acute appendicitis in the elderly. *J. Am. Board Fam. Pract.* 1996; 9: 75-8.
39. Terasawa, T. Blakemore, C.C., Bent, S, and Kohlwes, R.J. Systematic review: computed tomography and ultrasonography to detect acute appendicitis in adults and adulescents. *Ann. Intern. Med.* 2004; 141: 537-46.
40. Flum, D.R., McClure, T.D., Morris. A. and Koepsell, T. Misdiagnosis of appendicitis and the use of diagnostic imaging. *J. Am. Coll. Surgeons.* 2005; 201: 933.
41. Rao, P. M., Rhea, J.T., Novelline, R. A., Mostafavi, A. A., McCabe, C.J., et al. Effect of computed tomography of the appendix on treatment of patients and on use of hospital resources. *N. Engl. J. Med.* 1998; 338: 141-6.
42. Styrud, J. Erikson, S., Nilsson, I., Ahlberg,G., Haapeniemi, S., Niuvius, G., Rexs, L., Badume, I., Grandstom, L. Appendicectomy versus antibiotic treatment in acute appendicitis. A prospective multicenter randomized controlled trial. *World J Surg* 2006; 30: 1033.
43. Temple, C.L., Hutchcroft, S.A. and Temple, W.J. The natural history of appendicitis in adults: a prospective study. *Ann Surg* 1995; 221: 278-81.

Chapter 6
Peptic Ulcer Disease

E. Q. Archampong

Introduction

Nothing short of a revolution has characterized our understanding of the aetiology, pathogenesis and management of peptic ulcer disease over the past century and the burning issue that arises is how far this has influenced the outcome of current management of the disease. The decline of the acid dogma,[1,2] "no acid, no ulcer", which had given rise to decades of dominance of surgical interventions (partial gastrectomies, various forms of vagotomy), was succeeded by short term antibiotic regimes aimed at elimination of *helicobacter pylori* infection; this ensued following the demonstration that *H. pylori* is a primary factor in the pathogenesis of peptic ulcer disease by Warren and Marshall[3,4,] for which they were awarded the Nobel Prize for Medicine and Physiology in 2005. Furthermore non-steroidal anti-inflammatory drugs (NSAIDS) and low-dose asprin are currently increasingly associated with peptic ulcer disease in *H. pylori* negative individuals. This article attempts to review the current practice in West Africa in the management of the various forms of peptic ulcer disease, i.e. duodenal, gastric ulcers, gastro-esophageal reflux (GOERD), and its outcome.

Pathogenesis of Peptic Ulcer Disease

This remains complex but basically, there is imbalance of aggressive gastric luminal agents, mainly acid and the digestive enzyme pepsin, and the defensive mucosal barrier function; so acid secretion still plays an important role. However a whole range of environmental and host factors contribute to ulcerogenesis by increasing acid or pepsin secretion or through impairment of gastric mucosal barrier function.[2,5,6]

Among the former, tobacco use and alcoholism and drug agents have been cited but apart from NSAID use, none of these have been specifically backed by research data.[2] Although emotional stress is frequently blamed for ulcerogenesis, there is more objective support for severe organic stress from sepsis, burns and head or cerebral injuries.[7,8]

The Influence of H. Pylori

Although there is a very strong epidemiological association between H. pylori infection and duodenal and gastric ulceration, the ultimate confirmation of H. pylori as the main cause has been the demonstration of permanent cure of peptic ulcers by the eradication of H. pylori infection.[9,10] The fact is that while more that 50 percent of the world's population is chronically infected with H. pylori (and the figure reaches 75 percent in developing countries), only 5-10 per cent of those so infected develop ulcers. It seems the pattern of histological gastritis induced is one of the main determining factors. Thus in patients with duodenal ulcer, density and severity of infection are greatest in the distal and antral region, sparing the acid-secreting body mucosa, while in gastric ulcer the inflammation affects the body and antral mucosa to a similar degree, leading to much reduced gastric acid secretion, because of the more severe involvement of the acid secreting mucosa of the body of the stomach. There are also factors such as ulcerogenic strains of H. pylori and genetic factors and their influence on gastric and duodenal metaplasia.

H. pylori infection impairs the negative feed-back regulation of gastrin release. Through its capacity for high urease activity, it not only protects the organism from the low gastric pH, but also prevents the D cells in the gastric mucosa from sensing the true level of gastric acidity, thus stimulating an inappropriate release of stematostatin (decrease) resulting in an increase in gastrin release, leading to excessive acid secretion[11]

One of the effects of excessive gastric acid secretion is development of metaplasia in the duodenal bulb, leading to islands of colonization of the duodenal mucosa, a phenomenon more often seen in gastric than duodenal mucosa. The inflamed metaplasic duodenal mucosa is more susceptible to ulceration with further acid exposure.

The mucosal inflammation generated in the gastric mucosa appears more severe, with induction of epithelium-derived cytokines, particularly interleukin,[8] interleukin 1[12] producing an influx of neutrophils, macrophages with release of lysosomal enzymes, leucotrines and reactive oxygen free radicals, which impair mucosal resistance, releasing a process of immunopathogenic ulcerogenesis. In this scenario, even the reduced acid environment in the gastric mucosa, vitiated by body and antral gastritis, succumbs readily to gastric ulcer.

The NSAID Factor in Ulcerogenesis

This was earlier attributed to topical injury through ion trapping and reduction of mucosa gel protective activity;[13] subsequently this was shown to be more likely through suppression of gastric prostaglandin synthesis. The demonstration of two isoforms of cyclo-oxygenase i.e. Cox 1 and Cox 2, with the latter (anti-prostaglandin) exerting a selective gastric mucosa-sparing anti-inflammatory action, gave credence to this, though it is recognised that this does not eliminate entirely gastroduodenal ulcers and their complications.

The question that arises is whether any interaction exists between *H. pylori* and NSAIDS in the genesis of gastroduodenal ulceration? A natural additive or synergistic ulcerogenic action would be expected, but the evidence to date remains controversial. There are reports that increases in *H. pylori* infection have no effect on ulcer risk in NSAID users.[14,15]

Diagnosis

This is made difficult and often problematic because of the paucity of abdominal symptoms and signs. Epigastric pain or discomfort associated with meals is the predominant symptom of uncomplicated peptic ulcer, often associated with other dyspeptic symptoms – bloating, fullness, early satiety and nausea. With duodenal ulcers the pain is characteristically worse in the fasting state e.g. overnight in the early hours, and promptly relieved by intake of food or acid neutralizing agents, such as milk or alkaline patent medicines. Some

30 percent of duodenal ulcer (DU) patients complain of heart burn and may have reflux oesophagitis. Gastric ulcers occur in older patients, 45 and above and symptoms classically start within half an hour of feeding, and are accompanied by vomiting which relieves the dyspepsia.

It is important to recognize that chronic peptic ulcer may adopt a cyclical or seasonal pattern, a form of periodicity. Both chronic duodenal and gastic ulcers may be asymptomatic. This is particularly true of NSAID-induced ulcers, for which upper gastrointestinal bleeding or perforation may be the first clinical intimation of peptic ulcer disease.

In presentation overall, the most frequent complication is bleeding, with the highest risk in individuals over 60. Perforation, which is classically free resulting in peritonitis or localizing, or as acute exacerbation of the ulcer, is next, and shows no age predilection. The incidence of peritonitis from peptic ulcer perforation has been on the increase in recent years in Ghana.[16] Penetration of ulcers into retroperitoneal organs (pancreas) or the posterior abdominal wall is much less frequent and is marked by constant severe pain. Among African patients, ulcer fibrosis leading to gastric outlet obstruction is still frequently encountered, notwithstanding widespread exhibition of ulcer management regimes.

The dyspepsia that leads to the diagnosis of gastric or duodenal ulcer may be indistinguishable from the presentation of gastro oesophageal reflux diseases (GOERD) and may be so distinguished by the accompanying heart burn, retrosternal pain, radiation of the pain between the shoulder blades, worsening of the pain by stooping or lying down and relief by sitting upright. Since this latter group of symptoms may not be admitted by the patient, it behoves clinicians to maintain a high sense of suspicion to confirm or rule out accompanying gastro oesophageal reflux disease.

Confirmation of the of diagnosis of peptic ulcer disease is usually made at upper gastrointestinal endoscopy, when there is a mucosal break of 5mm or more, covered with fibrin. The 5mm criterion is arbitrary but it often corresponds with the pathological criterion of penetration of the muscularis mucosae. The typical location of duodenal ulcer is in the bulb where gastric contents first impinge on the intestinal mucosa.

Ulceration in the more distal duodenum or jejunum raises suspicions of unusual underlying disease – Zollinger Ellison Syndromes or Crohn's disease. The site of predilection for gastric ulcers is the angulus of the lesser curve, but could be sited anywhere from the pylorus to the cardia and the further away from the site of predilection, the greater the suspicions of the innocence of the mucosal breach. Gastric ulcers are more variable in their size which bear no relation to malignant potential. Endoscopic diagnosis of peptic ulcer disease must always be complemented with biopsies of antral, body, fundus or any suspicious tissue close to the ulcerating mucosa for histological studies as well as detection of *H. pylori* infection by rapid urease tests.

Dyspepsia is such a common complaint that in young patients (under 50 years) it is considered good practice to side step the invasive endoscopic investigation by simply doing the C-urea breath test, CLO test or stool antigen test and treat with H. pylori eradication if positive. The rationale for this protocol is that symptoms in a high proportion of such young patients would be due to underlying ulcer diseases that would be cured by *H. pylori* eradication; this would be plausible in such young people in whom neoplasia is rare in the absence of the alarm symptoms – anorexia, weight loss and anaemia.

The high incidence of dyspepsia as a complaint among young Ghanaians and the high level of inappropriate referrals for oesophago-gastro-duodenocopy reported at the Korle Bu Teaching Hospital,[17] a worldwide phenomenon where ever there is open access to the service on offer-- would tend to validate the practice of treating early symptoms of dyspepsia symptomatically using antacids, and reserving the invasive endoscopic procedure for persistent symptoms which require specific diagnosis and targeted therapy.

It is clear that upper gastrointestinal endoscopy has superceded all diagnostic modalities in management of peptic ulcer disease. The place of contrast radiological procedures and gastric secretory tests is severely restricted. This calls for the provision of endoscopic services, especially in the developing world. Indeed, definitive treatment of peptic ulcer disease without endoscopy is seriously flawed.

Management

The dogma "no acid, no ulcer" focused development of conserv-ative therapies on control of acid secretion and mucosal defense mechanisms. The successful drugs inhibiting acid secretion were the H2 receptor antagonists which provided the environment to heal ulcers, but problems arose in keeping them healed in remission unless maintenance therapy was instituted. They were superseded by proton pump inhibitors (PPI), more potent in suppression of acid secretion, but still requiring maintenance dosing to keep recurrence at bay in remission.

Mucosal barrier reinforcement was applied particularly where NSAIDS or asprin constituted an active aetiological factor; the potent prostaglandin analogue, misoprostol, was the most frequently employed agent, but its application was limited by abdominal untoward effects. Sucralfate and bismulth salts also enhance muscosal repair.

Where *H. pylori* infection is established there is no doubt that treatment directed at *H. pylori* eradication is the most effective protocol, and this is achieved through a combination of acid-inhibiting therapy and antibiotics. The problem in recent times has been the increasing levels of antibiotic resistance evinced by various strains of H. pylori. The Maastricht consensus Report (see Table 6.1) has provided clear guide lines for prescription of agents. The first line triple therapy regime is Proton Pump inhibitor (PPI) and antibiotic combination (Esomeprazole 40mg, clarithromycin 500mg bd and amoxicillin 1G bd for 7-14 days).

H. pylori eradication is as effective in duodenal as gastric ulceration. In duodenal ulcer testing using non invasive measures (i.e. C- Urease Breath Test and stool antigen testing) can be relied on as surrogate maker confirming healing. In gastric ulcer on the other hand healing needs to be confirmed through endoscopic biopsies to avoid missing malignancies, even when the ulcer appears to be healing. For duodenal ulcers a 14 days eradication regime need not be followed by further PPI administration. In gastrc ulcers on the other hand PPI adminis-tration needs to be continued for 4-8 weeks.

The Maastricht Consensus on H. Pylori Eradication

Table 6.1   Helicobacter pylori eradication regimens

First-line options (7-14day s)

- In populations with less than 15-20 percent clarithromycin resistance and greater than 40 percent metronidazole resistance proton-pump inhibitor (PPI) standard dose, clarithromycin 2x500mg, and amoxicillin 2x1000 mg, all given twice a day;
- Less than 15-20 percent clarithromycine resistance and less than 40 percent metroinidazole resistance: PPI standard dose, clarithromycin 500mg, and metronidazole 400 mg or tinidazole 500 mg, all given twice a day In areas with high clarithromycin and metronidazole resistance bismuth containing quadruple therapy.

Second-line options (10-14 days)

- Bismuth-containing quadruple therapy gastrointestinal bleeding. *World Journal of Gastrointestinal Surgery,* 2011;3:89-100.
- PPI plus metronidazole and amoxicillin, if clarithromycine was used in first-line treatment (in Latin America and China, furazolidone 2-4x100mg is often preferred over metronidazole).

Rescue therapies (10-14 days)

- PPI twice a day plus amoxicillin 2x1000mg with either levofloxacin 2x250 (500) mg, or with rifabutin 2x150mg.

Treatment in NSAID Induced Ulcers

In developed countries where *H. pylori* infection is on the decline, NSAIDs and low-dose aspirin have come into sharp prominence as cause for peptic ulcer and its complications. In patients developing duodenal or gastric ulcer while receiving NSAIDs, some 90 percent heal within 8 weeks of standard H2 receptor antagonists (ranitidine 150 mg bd) provided the offending NSAIDs are withdrawn. Healing of gastric ulcers in particular is severely impaired when NSAID dosing continues. Some recent studies[18,19] have suggested that PPI (esomeperazole) might be better than ranitidine in healing gastric ulcer patients who continue dosing with NSAIDs, but no conclusive clinical trials of these agents are as yet available.

H. Pylori and NSAID Negative Ulcers

With the rising use of antimicrobial agents worldwide, it is becoming frequent even in developing countries to see patients with peptic ulcer disease who test H. pylori negative and persistently deny the use of NSAIDs for months. This is a special group of peptic ulcer patients, and it is expedient to ascertain the H. pylori and NSAID/asprin status of such patients by endoscopic biopsy and detailed history. They may turn out to have the Zollinger-Ellison syndrome, multiple endocrine adenopathy (MENS) or to have experienced exposure to high dose upper abdominal radiotherapy. High dose PPI therapy has virtually replaced total gastrectomy in such cases where the offending gastrinoma cannot be located.

There are still some gastric and duodenal ulcers for which no recognized underlying aetiological agency is discernable. Some of these may be attributable to rebound acid secretion that results from withdrawal of PPI therapy. For such patients, higher doses still of PPI might be needed since it is now realised that the inhibitory effects of PPI are less in individuals without H. pylori infection.[20] The other form of peptic ulcer of undetermined orgin is stress ulcer, originally described by Cushing in patients with cerebral trauma and patients with severe burns, sepsis, multiple organ dysfunction and patients requiring ventillatory support. The necessary stress ulcer prophylaxis can be undertaken with either PPI or H2 – receptor antagonists, since no clear-cut difference in benefit, morbidity or mortality has been demonstrated by recent studies.[21]

Surgical Management of Peptic Ulcer Disease

The de-escalation of surgical intervention noted in the latter decades of the 20th century has become almost a trickle at the beginning of the

21st. Most cases of duodenal ulcer respond to conservative triple or quadruple therapy.

The only indications for surgical intervention in uncomplicated ulcers are chronicity, the decision on which may turn out to be parlous, or surgical complications mostly presenting as emergencies. Ulcers become refractory to conservative therapy because they are *H. pylori* negative, unrelated to NSAID or asprin use, or on account of failure of *H. pylori* eradication. Few cases can be attributed to failure of lifestyle modification that should complement any treatment regime. The current first-line recommendation for such duodenal ulcers is truncal vagotomy with drainage (pyloroplasty or gastro-jeunostomy). The procedure is associated with a number of troublesome complications – dumping, diarrhoea, stetorrhoea enterogastric reflux, and iron deficiency anaemia. Most of these improve with time and the ulcer recurrence rate, at 5-10 percent in 10 years, is tolerable.

The alternative operation for chronicity is highly selective or proximal gastric vagotomy (HSV, PGV) without drainage. The ulcer recurrence rate is however rather high i.e. 25 percent in 5 years and more than 40 percent in 15 years. This is a serious draw back, inspite of the low level of post vagotomy symptoms, less than 5 percent. The operation is hardly practised in recent years. Vagotomy and antrectomy (with gastro-duodenal anastomosis) has lower incidence of complications compared with partial gastrectomy (Polya or Bilroth II) and the mortality less than 1 percent, but the ulcer recurrence rate may be quite high in the longer term. Both operations are now resorted to in highly recalcitrant duodenal ulcers.

Gastric outlet obstruction from cicatrisation and oedema is a common and early complication of duodenal ulceration in Africa and the Indian subcontinent as opposed to Western communities, where the incidence is lower. It responds promptly to fluids and electrolyte resuscitation and may resolve with triple ulcer therapy where oedema is the predominating pathology presenting. Excessive fibrosis nearly always demands operative intervention on resuscitation, and the procedure of choice is truncal vagotomy and gastrojejunostomy. The outcome is good where the lesion results from duodenal ulcer cicatrisation.

Duodenal ulcer perforations nearly always require surgical intervention on resuscitation and most patients do well on simple closure, buttressed with a pad of omentum. It is essential to complement surgical intervention with a standard course of first-line triple therapy. Patients who have protracted history of peptic ulceration, punctuated by previous repeated episodes of medical therapy, may be considered for definitive curative ulcer surgery, i.e. vagotomy and drainage, providing they present within a few hours of perforation. Perforations however tend to present rather late in West African communities, sometimes several days after the incident.[16] This of course worsens the prognosis and discourages attempts at definitive curative ulcer surgery.

Bleeding ulcers usually respond to conservative measures with volume replacement, triple therapy and endoscopic manipulations for local arrest of the haemorrhage, including mucosal injections of saline, adrenaline, polidocanol and mucosal thermocoagulation and in difficult cases arterial embolisation.[22] Surgical intervention is indicated in older patients (over 50 year old) with cardiovascular instability and the standard procedure is control of haemorrhage by under running of the bleeding vessel.

The indications for surgical intervention in gastric ulcers have over time crystalised out: an ulcer that does not show endoscopic evidence of complete or at least 50 percent healing in four weeks must be considered for surgical therapy, if there is no definitive healing on a further two-week period of observation. Persistent symptoms in spite of repeated *H. pylori* eradication (failed medical therapy), atypically placed ulcers e.g. greater curve ulcers must also be treated surgically on account of the high malignant potential of these ulcers.

The procedure of choice is a hemi- or two-thirds distal gastric resection, excising the area of chronic atrophic gastritis with a gastroduodenal reconstruction. This way the areas of further ulceration and possible malignancy are eliminated. The results are good with a recurrence rate of 1-3 percent and 5-10 percent incidence of mild post-gastrectomy symptoms. The alternative procedure is truncal vagotomy with excision of the ulcer to exclude malignancy.

The operation is simpler with fewer complications, but the recurrence rate is high, about 10-15 percent of individuals. Surgical resection is preferred in patients presenting with acute complications – perforation, obstruction – gastric outlet obstruction.

Conclusion

The management of peptic ulcer disease has become increasingly conservative in recent decades. Control of the disease within communities has been effective, but for problems of compliance on account of lack of access to the necessary drugs in the community. Patients with complications requiring surgical intervention tend to present late, with gross pathological changes which are often attended by poor outcome. Peptic ulcer disease is essentially a benign condition, and should be attended by favourable outcome, as has happened in the cases amenable to conservative management with drugs. It needs to be emphasized that complications are attended by poorer outcomes because of emergent surgery especially in the aged. Early diagnosis and intensification of medical therapy with a view to reducing the incidence of complications should be the way forward.

References

1. Gustafson J., and Welling D. No-Acid No Ulcer 100 years later. A Review of the History of Peptic Ulcer Disease *Journal of American College of Surgeons* 210: 110-116.
2. Malferheiner., P., Chan, FKL., Mccoll,E.L. Seminar, Peptic Ulcer Disease *Lancet* 2009 374: 1449-1461.
3. Warren, J.R., and Marshal,l B. Unidentified curved bacilli on gastric epithelium in active chronic gastritis, *Lancet* 1983: 321: 1273-1275
4. Marshal, B.J. and Warrant, J.R. Unidentified curved bacilli in the stomach of patients with gastritis and peptic ulceration. *Lancet,* 1984 323: 1311-1315.
5. Davenport, H.N. Salicylate damage to the gastric mucosal barrier. *New England Journal of Medicine*, 1967; 276: 130-7 – 1312.
6. Grossman, M.I. Abnormalities of acid secretion in patients with duodenal ulcer. *Gastroenterology.*, 1978; 75: 524-526.
7. Alain, B.B. and Wang, Y.J. Cushing's ulcer in traumatic brain injury. *Clinical Journal Traumatol,* 2008; 11: 114-119.

8.   Gratrix, A.P., Enright, S.M.and O' Beirne, H.A. A survey of stress prophylaxis in intensive care units in the *U.K. Anaesthesia,* 2007; 62: 421-422.

9.   Ravws, E.A.J. and Tytgat, G.N.J. Cure of duodenal ulcer associated with eradication of H. pylori, *Lancet,* 1990 335: 1233-1235.

10. Malfertheinerm P., Leodolter, A. and Peitz, U. Cure of H. pylori associated ulcer disease through eradication. *Baillieres Best Prac. Res. Clin. Gastroenterology,* 2000; 14:119-132.

11. Graham, D.Y. Go, M.E., Lew, C.I.M., Genta, R.M., Rechfeld, J.F. H pylori infection and exaggerated gastrin release. Effects of inflammation and progastrin processing. *Scand J. Gastroenterology,* 1993: 28 690-694.

12. Dixon, M.F. Patterns of inflammation linked to ulcer disease. *Baillieres Best Pract Respiratory Clinical Gastroenterol, 2000: 14: 27-449.*

13. Davenport, H.W. Gastric mucosal haemorrhage in dogs. Effects of acid, asprin and alcohol. *Gastroenterology,* 1969 56: 439-449.

14. Labenz, J., Blum, A.l. and Bolten, W. W. et al. Primary prevention of diclofenac associated ulcers and dyspepsia by omeperazole or triple therapy in H. pylori positive patients a randomized double blind placebo controlled clinical trial. *Gut,* 2002; 51: 329-335.

15. Chan, F.K., Hung, L.C., Suen, B.Y. et al Celecoxibversus diclofenac plus omeperazole in high risk arthritis patients results of a randomized double blind trial. *Gastroenterology,* 2004;127: 1038-1043.

16. Dakubo, J.C.B., Naaeder, S.B. and Clegg-Lamptey, J.N. Gastroduoenal peptic ulcer perforation. *East African Medical Journal,* 2009;100-109.

17. Tachi, K. and Nkrumah, K.N. Appropriateness and Diagnostic Yield of Referrals for Oesophago-gastro-duodenoscopy at the Korle-Bu Teaching Hospital. *West African Journal of Medicine,* 2011;30:158-16.

18. Yeomans, N.O., Svedberg, L.E. and Neasdal, J. Is ranitidine therapy sufficient for healing peptic ulcers associated with non-steroidal anti inflammatory drug use. *Int. Journal Clinical Pract.* 2006; 60 1401-1407.

19. Goldstein, J.L., Johanso, J.F., Hawkey, C.J., Suchover, L.J.and Brown K.A. Clinical Trial: healing of NSA associated gastric ulcers in patients continuing NSAID therapy, a randomized study comparing ranitidine omeperazole. *Aliment Pharmacol Ther.* 2007 26: 1101-1111.

20. Verdu, E.F., Armstrong, D., Frazer, R. et al. Effect of H pylori status on intragastric pH during treatment with omeperazole. *Gut,* 1995 36: 539-543.

21.	Kahn, J.M., Doctor, J.N.and Rubenfeld, G.D. Stress ulcer prophylaxis in mechanically ventilated patients: integrating evidence and judgment using a decision analysis. *Intensive Care Med.* 2006 32: 1151-1158.
22.	Loffroy, R.F., Abuaalsaud, B.A., Lin, M.B. and Rao, P.P. Recent advances in endovascular technique for management of acute non varieal upper gastrointestinal bleeding 2011 *World Journal of Gastrointestinal Surgery,* 2011; 3:89-100.

Chapter 7
Gastrointestinal Stromal Tumours (GIST)

B. Baako

Epidemiology

GIST is the commonest mesenchymal neoplasm of the gastrointestinal tract. European incidence[1] per annum has been estimated at 10-20/ million and a prevalence of 129/million. Malignant transformation is seen in 20-30 percent of newly diagnosed cases per year. One surgical unit in Korle Bu Teaching Hospital saw 8 cases over a 6-year period (unpublished data) with only one case less than 5cm in the widest diameter. It is seen commonly in the over 50 years age group with a median between 55 and 65 years [2]. The gender preference in not settled, but there may be a slight male preponderance. Ethnicity, race, geographical location, and environmental factors are not known to influence the incidence. Rarely, GISTs may arise from other organs, extragastro intestinal GIST (eGIST). This may be from the mesentery, omentum, and the peritoneal surface. Cases have been reported arising from the gall bladder, liver, pancreas and the urinary bladder.

Distribution of GISTs in the GIT

Oesophagus	Stomach	Duodenum and Small Intestine	Colon and Rectum
5%	50-60%	30-40%	5%

GIST may occur in the paediatric age group but the incidence is not known. Familial GIST - an autosomal dominant trait was described in 1998.[3] There are germ line mutations in addition to kit mutation. Neurofibromatosis (von Recklinghausen disease), extra-adrenal para-ganglionoma and oesophageal leiomyoma (Carney triad) are associated with gastric GISTs .[4]

Histopathology (pathogenesis)

GISTs are mesenchymal tumours that show differentiation towards the Carjal cells or their progenitor stem-cells. The main event is the mutation of the kit CD117 or the PDGFRA genes. This then promotes the uncontrolled activation of the protein kinase site to produce tumour protein thus enhancing cell proliferation and tumour growth[5]. Furthermore, approximately 50 percent to 70 percent of GISTS, especially of the small bowel, express the CD34 on the cell surface. Secondary mutations may occur during treatment with tyrosine kinase inhibitors resulting in drug resistance 960[6]. The site and type of mutation may affect prognosis. Gastric GIST arising from deletion behave more aggressively than those from duplication. Kit mutations affecting codons 557-558 also have unfavourable outcomes. GISTs that do not have KIT mutations, PDGFRA mutations, (20 to 30 percent gastric) often have primary resistance to imatinib.

Histologically there are the spindle, epithelioid and the mixed epitheliod and spindle cell types. Site specific GISTs tend to have variations in cell types. Stomach GISTs are more epithelioid than spindle cells. Intestinal ones have more spindle cells.

Prognosis

Unlike most malignancies, GISTs have no grading/staging systems. The risk of recurrence of completely excised GIST with healthy margins is determined/predicted by the mitotic rate/50hpf, tumour size and tumour site.[7]

Risk group	Mitotic rate	Tumour size (cm)
Very low	< 5	< 2
Low	< 5	2-5
Intermediate	6-10	< 5
High	> 5	> 5
	Any	>10
	>10	any

Tumours of similar size and mitotic index have poorer prognosis if in the small bowel than in the stomach. Poor performance status, high white cell count with absolute neutrophilia and low haemoglobin are clinical indicators of poor prognosis.

Distribution of GISTs in gastrointestinal tract

Oesophageal GISTs occur most commonly in the distal third and constitute only 5 percent of all GISTs. Most are greater than 5cm in diameter. The commonest site is the stomach (70 percent) and can grow exophytically up to more than 40cm in diameter. They commonly show epithelioid cell type with better prognosis. Duodenal GISTs, 4 to 5 percent of all GISTs, tend to show histologically a spindle cell differentiation with poorer prognosis. Like the duodenal type, the other small bowel GISTs are morphologically spindle cell type with similar prognosis.

Clinical diagnosis

Most GISTs present with abdominal mass, GIT bleeding with anaemia, or obstructive bowel symptoms. Some present with nonspecific symptoms, and others are found incidentally while investigating for other conditions by endoscopy, radiological imaging or even laparotomy for other reasons. Those incidental findings are usually small in size.

CT scan of the abdomen and pelvis shows an inhomogeneously enhanced mass lesion. They may show polypoid exophytic or endophytic growth although the swellings are generally centered on the bowel wall. Lymph nodes are rarely involved. There may be liver secondaries and/or serosal nodules. Gastric lesions are visualised as submucosal protruberances with central necrosis on endoscopy. Endoscopic US may be helpful. Biopsy for histological confirmation of the diagnosis may not be necessary before surgical intervention for fear of spillage. In those cases that will need neoadjuvant treatment, tissue diagnosis is important to exclude lymphomas. Core biopsies are taken under image guidance, i.e. US or CT guided.

Treatment of GISTs

There are two modalities of treatment, surgery and the tyrosine kinase inhibitors independently or in combination.

The principle of surgical treatment is total removal of the tumour (Figure 7.1) with clear margins (histological clear margins) avoiding intra-peritoneal rupture or bleeding.[8,9] The literature reports 42 percent 5 years overall survival for clear margins in contrast to 9 percent overall survival for the same period for none-clear margins. Intra peritoneal leakage is associated with high local recurrence of up to 100 percent. Where the tumour is attached to surrounding structures en block dissection is advised. Should these conditions not be satisfied, adjuvant tyrosine kinase inhibitor is indicated. Small or intermediate tumours (< 5cm) can be excised laparoscopically.

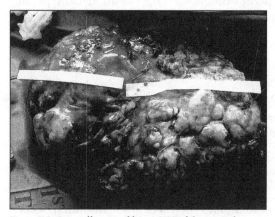

Figure 7.1: Surgically excised large GIST of the stomach

Neoadjuvant therapy with tyrosine kinase inhibitors

Indications include inoperable tumour, avoidance of mutilating surgery, downstaging of the tumour to facilitate resection and reduce the possibility of intra-operative tumour rupture or bleeding with its consequent poor outcomes. The wild type kit gene and unfavourable mutations in the KIT or PDGFRA do not respond to imatinib treatment. PET/CT scans are therefore performed at regular intervals (most authors after one month) to assess response and to put in place the necessary surgical intervention if indicated. Some also develop secondary resistance to the drug. It is advised that responders be operated on within the first 6-12 (others suggest 3-4) months from the start of therapy[10] although rectal and oesophageal lesions may be delayed provided they continue to respond to the tyrosine kinase inhibitors.

Adjuvant therapy

After complete surgical resection of GISTs, the 5-year overall survival (OS) has been reported as 54 percent. In metastatic disease the mean survival was 19 months. The American College of Surgeons Oncology Group have shown that imatinib treatment prolonged recurrence free survival and improved OS after complete surgical resection of KIT positive GISTs of high risk of recurrence (>10cm, tumour rupture, <5cm but with mets). In their study, exon 11 mutations had 62 percent 3-year disease-free survival, PDGFRA mutant patients had 90 percent 3-year disease free survival and 77 percent 3-year disease-free survival in patients without detectable mutation.[11]

Duration of imatinib treatment of GIST is yet to be determined. Some studies reported relapse, 6 months after 1 year and 3 years treatment with the tyrosine kinase inhibitors were stopped. Drug resistance may also develop.

The factors that determine who receives tyrosine kinase inhibitors include tumour size, mitotic index, mutation type and site and the quality of the surgery performed.

The practice guideline in the management of GISTs in early stages is complete surgical resection with clear margins plus adjuvant tyrosine kinase inhibitors in those cases of increased risk of local recurrence.

References

1. Nilsson, B. Bumming, P., Meis-Kindblom, J. Gastrointestinal stomal tumours: the incidence, prevalence, clinical course, and prognostication in the pre-imatinib mesylate era – a population based study in Western Sweden: *Cancer* 2005; 103: 821-82.

2. Goettsch, W.G., Bos, S.D., Breekfeldt-Postma, N. (2005) Incidence of gastrointestinal stromal tumours is underestimated: results of a nationwide study: *Eur J Cancer,* 41 (18) 2868-2872.

3.   Nishida, T., Hibota, S., Taniguchi, M. et al. (1998) Familial gastroin-
      testinal stromal tumours with gemline mutation of the KIT gene: *Nat
      Genet* 19 (4) 323-324.

4.   Carney, J.A., Sheps, S.G., Go, V.L. and Gordon, H. (1977). The triad
      of gastric leiomyoma, functioning extra-adrenal paraganglioma and
      pulmonary chondroma: *N Eng J Med* 296 (26): 1517-1518.

5.   Hirota, S., Isozaki., K. Moriyama. et al. (1998). Gain of function
      mutations of c-kit in human gastrointestinal stromal tumours. *Science*
      279 (5350):577-580.

6.   DeMatteo, R.P., Lewis, J.J., Leung, D, et al. (2000). Two hundred
      gastrointestinal stromal tumours: recurrence patterns and prognostic
      factors for survival: *Ann Surg.* 231 (1) 51-58.

7.   Pierie, J.P., Choudry, U., Muzikansky, A. et al. The effect of surgery and
      grade on outcome of gastrointestinal stromal tumours. *Arch Surg.* 136
      (4) 383-389.

8.   Hohenberger, P., Ronellenfltsch, U., Oladeji., O. et al. (2010). Pattern
      of recurrence in patients with ruptured primary gastrointestinal
      tumours. *Br J Surg,* 97(12) 1854-1859).

9.   Miettinan, M. and Lasota, J. (2006) Gastrointestinal stromal tumours:
      pathology and prognosis at different sites. *Semin Diagn Pathol* 23(2)
      70-83.

10.   Eisenberg, B.L. and Smith, K.D. (2011). Adjuvant and neoadjuvant
      therapy for primary gastrointestinal stromal tumours: *Cancer
      Chemother Pharmaco* 67 (suppl 1).

11.   DeMatteo, R.P., Owzar, K., Antonescu, C.R. et al. (2008): Efficacy of
      adjuvant imatinib mesylate following complete resection of localized
      primary GIST at high risk of recurrence: The US Intergroup phaseII
      trial ACOSOG 2 900: *Gastrointestinal cancers symposium* 2008.

Chapter 8
Malignant Gastric Neoplasms; Hope for the Future
N.A. Adu-Aryee

Introduction

Gastric cancers are a diverse group of cancers which are known to have a poor prognosis worldwide except in Japan and Korea.[1]

The predominant cancer type worldwide is the adenocarcinoma arising from mucosa and forms 90 percent of all gastric neoplasms. The two main variants are the diffuse and intestinal types with different presentations and prognosis.[2]

Lesions also arise from lymphoid tissues which are not native to the stomach but are present because of chronic irritation.

The main irritant which is also shared with the adenocarcinoma sub-group is the relatively newly found organism *Helicobacter pylori* *(H pylori)*.[3]

In lymphoid neoplasms the lesions are known as Mucosa Associated Lymphoid Tissue (MALT) Lymphomas.[4]

The muscle layer also contributes its share of malignancy through the interstitial cells of Cajal which are the intrinsic pacemaker cells of the stomach. The resulting tumours formerly thought to be leiomyosarcomas (arising from smooth muscle) are now referred to as stromal tumours hence the term Gastro-Intestinal Stromal Tumours, or GISTs.[5]

Prognosis for adenocarcinomas of the stomach have been considered as poor except in Japan where the disease is considered a public health problem and so early detection and radical surgery for early lesions give survival rates of over 90 percent.[6] This has not been duplicated in other places leading to research into supplementary forms of treatment, some of which have shown statistically significant improvements in survival rates. These modalities include peri-operative chemotherapy[7] and postoperative chemoradiation[8] and in some cases targeted therapies against Human Epidermal Receptor II where this is over-expressed.[9]

The presence of *H pylori* in the aetiology of MALT lymphomas also lends itself to a therapeutic option of organism eradication in treatment of this condition as part of the armamentarium.[10]

The GISTs are the group which have been in the forefront of research, targeted treatments for tyrosine kinase inhibitors showing the way.[11] There are also a tiny subset of neuroendocrine tumours which are apparently quite chemosensitive.

This review will focus on the experience with adenocarcinomas within the Korle Bu Teaching Hospital(KBTH).

Adenocarcinomas of the stomach

Known to be quite aggressive, these lesions have been known to be detected only when symptomatic and advanced in nature except for countries with early detection or screening policies.

The worldwide incidence is not known but in Europe 159,900 cases were reported in 2006 with 118,200 deaths recorded.[12]

In the USA, 38,780 upper gastrointestinal tumours are projected to occur in 2012, of which 25,610 patients are expected to die.[13]

Operating theatre records for KBTH in Accra suggest that in 2010, seven patients had partial gastrectomies with three having palliative bypasses for obstruction. In 2011, there were eight gastric resections with three bypasses. These figures suggest that most of the cases are still fairly advanced (Figure 8.1) making curative surgery next to impossible.

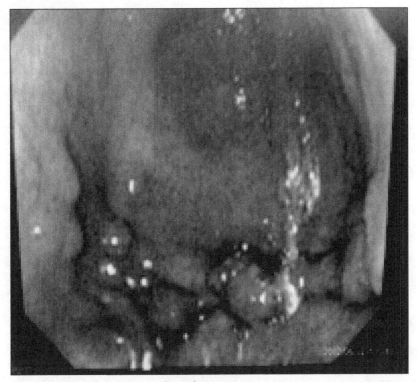

Figure 8.1: Advanced gastric cancer observed at gastroscopy

Mortality rates for gastric cancers have been known to be high and dependent on stage of occurrence or presentation of the lesions.

The incidence worldwide is generally thought to be declining. This has been attributed to changes in food storage patterns and the use of frozen foods rather than salted or pickled foods. Improvements in water supply have also been cited.

In Ghana Darko et al.1996 found a significant incidence of H Pylori in gastric pathology including tumours.[14] Unpublished data by Archampong, T. (personal communication) in Accra also correlate this finding.

Other factors like ingestion of well-done red meat, drinking green tea and familial disease patterns have been cited.

The worrying trend however is a relative increase in the number of proximal as opposed to distal tumours in the Western world or in low-risk areas.[15] The implications of having more proximal tumours which seem to behave like distal oesophageal tumours is a relatively poorer prognosis with more extensive surgical procedures and more physiologic stress on the patient. This increase in proximal tumours has been linked to increasing obesity in the general populace together with an increase in the incidence of reflux oesophagitis.[15,16] The true reason for these changes in epidemiology is not known.

Unpublished endoscopy suite figures for the KBTH for 2010 and 2011 give total endoscopic cancer rates of 47 out of 1,066 and 68 out of 2,168 upper gastrointestinal endoscopies done. Proximal to distal tumour ratios of 30 to 17 (2:1) and 41 to 27(1.5:1) were also documented for the two years in question. This suggests that the trend of higher ratios of distal to proximal tumours has not occurred yet in Ghana.

Worldwide the male-to-female ratio of gastric cancer of 2:1 seems to have been maintained as the figures for 2010 and 2011 in the Korle Bu Hospital series remained approximately 2:1 and 1.5:1 respectively.[17]

The major disappointment is in the fact that only one of all the diagnoses made clinically on endoscopic findings in the Korle Bu data was considered an early gastric cancer.

This is in keeping with worldwide rates out of Japan and south east Asia where the early detection rates are higher because of screening programmes.

The mean age for 2010 was 64 years while 2011 had 57 years as a mean age.[17] Here again the worldwide peak age incidence of 6th to 7th decade of life is maintained. Work done by Dakubo and also by Tachi on appropriateness of referrals for upper GI endoscopy also suggested most cases found were over 50 years old.[18,19]

Patients seen in the hospital had two main modalities of treatment: surgery and chemotherapy.

Surgery was mainly palliative in most cases. Addition of chemotherapy to the hospital's treatment schedules was the main improvement in quality of service offered to patients. The trial of perioperative chemotherapy and the postoperative chemoradiation trial improved outcomes in the Western world and also offered hope to Ghanaian patients although statistically insignificant gains were recorded.

A review of histologically confirmed gastric cancer cases seen between 2004 and 2008 at the Oncology Unit of Korle Bu Teaching Hospital was done. Twenty-seven cases were reviewed.

The retrospective data was analyzed for age and sex distribution, tumour type, location and outcomes to chemotherapy were made including toxicity profiles of drugs used.

In this series the male-to-female ratio was 3:1 with an age range of 24 to 84 years, the mean being 54 years. Fifteen of these patients (53 percent) had locally advanced disease, 12(42 percent) had metastatic disease and 1 had local recurrence.

Various combinations of chemotherapy were used, the main determinant being cost. Patients who had monotherapy with capecitabine were either elderly or frail. Patient tolerance of this regimen was good with few breaks between cycles. Capecitabine was also combined with cisplatin in 10 patients preoperatively but the toxicity rates were higher.

Seven of the patients had concurrent radiotherapy with resolution of symptomatic bleeding.

This series is hampered by lack of mortality data as it sought to look mainly at toxicity profiles.

Opportunities exist for further research into the characteristics of gastric tumours in Ghana and the prognostic features of these tumours.

Conclusion

The results suggest that with more aggressive adjuvant treatment, hopes of cure for patients with this distressing condition are improved. In addition research into the incidence of HER II receptor positivity may offer additional targets for treatment with hopes of better outcomes.

Research is also ongoing into less toxic forms of chemotherapeutic regimens with similar efficacy to proven regimens. Genetic tumour profiling with respect to prediction of response to various treatment regimens is also gaining ground in the hope of avoiding the subjection of patients to toxic regimens which may not be effective.

References

1. Kamangar, F., Dores, G.M. and Anderson, W.F. G.M. Patterns of cancer incidence, mortality, and prevalence across five continents: defining priorities to reduce cancer disparities in different geographic regions of the world. *Journal of clinical oncology* : official journal of the American Society of Clinical Oncology, 2006. 24(14): p. 2137-50.

2. Roder, D.M., The epidemiology of gastric cancer. *Gastric cancer* : official journal of the International Gastric Cancer Association and the Japanese Gastric Cancer Association, 2002. 5: p. 5-11.

3. Atherton, J.C., The pathogenesis of Helicobacter pylori-induced gastro-duodenal diseases. *Annual review of pathology,* 2006. 1: p. 63-96.

4. Parsonnet, J., Hansen, S. Rodriguez, L. Helicobacter pylori infection and gastric lymphoma. *The New England journal of medicine,* 1994. 330(18): p. 1267-71.

5. Miettinen, M. and J. Lasota. Gastrointestinal stromal tumors: pathology and prognosis at different sites. *Seminars in diagnostic pathology*, 2006. 23(2): p. 70-83.

6. Overvad, K., Aoki, K., Hayakawa, N., Kurihar, M, Suzuki, S, eds. Death rates for malignant neoplasms for selected sites by sex and five-year age group in 33 countries. 1953-57 to 1983-87. Nagoya, Japan. The University of Nagoya Coop Press, 1992, 560 pages. *Scandinavian Journal of Public Health Scandinavian Journal of Public Health,* 1993. 21(1): p. 59-60.

7. Cunningham, D., Allum, W. H. and Stenning, S. P., Perioperative chemotherapy versus surgery alone for resectable gastroesophageal cancer. *The New England journal of medicine,* 2006. **355**(1): p. 11-20.

8. Macdonald, J.S., Smalley, S.R. and Benedetti,J., Chemoradiotherapy after Surgery Compared with Surgery Alone for Adenocarcinoma of the Stomach or Gastroesophageal Junction. *New England Journal of Medicine,* 2001. 345(10): p. 725-730.

9. Bang, Y.-J., Van Cutsen, E. and Feyereisslova, A. Trastuzumab in combination with chemotherapy versus chemotherapy alone for treatment of HER2-positive advanced gastric or gastro-oesophageal junction cancer (ToGA): a phase 3, open-label, randomised controlled trial. *The Lancet.* 376(9742): p. 687-697.

10. Lehours, P. and F. Mégraud. Helicobacter pylori infection and gastric MALT lymphoma. *Roczniki Akademii Medycznej w Bialymstoku* (1995), 2005. 50: p. 54-61.

11. Joensuu, H., Treatment of inoperable gastrointestinal stromal tumor (GIST) with Imatinib (Glivec, Gleevec). *Medizinische Klinik* (Munich, Germany : 1983), 2002. 97 Suppl 1: p. 28-30.

12. Ferlay, J., Autier, P., and Buniol,M., Estimates of the cancer incidence and mortality in Europe in 2006. *Annals of Oncology,* 2007. 18(3): p. 581-592.

13. Siegel, R., D. Naishadham, and A. Jemal, Cancer statistics, 2012. CA: *A Cancer Journal for Clinicians.* 62(1): p. 10-29.

14. Baako, B.N. and R. Darko, Incidence of Helicobacter pylori infection in Ghanaian patients with dyspeptic symptoms referred for upper gastrointestinal endoscopy. *West African journal of medicine,* 1996. 15(4); 223–27

15. Correa, P. and V.W. Chen, Gastric cancer. *Cancer surveys,* 1994. 19-20: p. 19-20.

16. Crew, K.D. and A.I. Neugut, Epidemiology of gastric cancer. World Journal of Gastroenterology : *WJG,* 2006. 12(3): p. 354-62.

17. Sipponen, P. and P. Correa, Delayed rise in incidence of gastric cancer in females results in unique sex ratio (M/F) pattern: etiologic hypothesis. *Gastric Cancer,* 2002. 5(4): p. 213-219.

18. Dakubo, J.C.N., Clegg-Lamptey, J. and Sowah, P. Appropriateness of Referrals for Upper Gastrointestinal Endoscopy. *West African Journal of Medicine* 2011. 30(5); 342–47.

19. Tachi, K. and Nkrumah, K.N. Appropriateness and Diagnostic Yield of Referrals for Oesophagogastroduodenoscopy at the Korle Bu Teaching Hospital. *West African Journal of Medicine* 2011 .30(3); 158–163.

Chapter 9
Management of Upper Gastrointestinal Bleeding

E. Q. Archampong.

Introduction

Upper gastrointestinal bleeding (UGIB) is usually an acute emergency which is defined as bleeding originating from the gastro-intestinal tract, proximal to the ligament of Treitz and made manifest by the symptoms of haematemesis and or melaena. Presentation is however not always clear cut and the bleeding may take unusual forms that may not be readily distinguishable from haemorrhage from lower reaches of the bowel. The approach to the control of the latter category of bleeding differs in several significant respects, and is therefore tackled in a subsequent paper; its consideration is nonetheless less essential in the initial assessment of all forms of gastrointestinal haemorrhage.

This presentation focuses on the current management of the principal causes of upper gastrointestinal haemorrhage in our practice emphasizing the need for urgent accurate assessment, patient triage and resuscitation, diagnosis and concerted action to influence outcome.

Epidemiology

The relative frequency of causes of upper GI bleeding varies in different regions of the world. In most parts of Africa, chronic peptic ulceration[1] (chronic duodenal and gastric ulcer (Du/Gv: 60/10) accounts for 50-90 per cent of cases. Notable exceptions to this are some East and Central African countries - Tanzania, Zimbabwe, Kenya - where oesophageal varices constitute a more common cause of bleeding than chronic peptic ulceration[8].

In Accra over a period of two years, some 552 cases of haematemesis and melaena referred to the endoscopy centre showed the following aetiological spread and symptomatology (Tables 9.1 and 9.2).

Clearly these are not population-based figures; the availability of the endoscopic expertise may have attracted to the centre a disproportionate number of bleeding cases. There is also a preponderance of bleeding from oesophageal and gastric varices, amounting to 30 percent, almost equal to the figures for combined gastric and duodenal ulcers, and almost approaching the pattern in East and Central Africa. Whether this is a reflection of latent high prevalence of subacute hepatic disease in the population or a selection phenomenon, occasioned by the location of the endoscopy centre, needs to be established by a purpose-designed and appropriately powered prospective study.

Notwithstanding the geographical variation in the causes of UGIB, in terms of frequency, in West Africa, as elsewhere, three categories are discernable.[1]

The common or major causes: duodenal/gastric ulcers and stress ulcers (including gastritis mucosal erosions) and oesophageal varices. The less common: oesophagitis (GORD) Mallory-Weiss Syndrome, benign and malignant tumours of the oesophagus, stomach and duodenum, and the rare group: invading pancreatic tumours aorto-enteric fistulae, blood dyscrasias hereditary telangiectasias angiodysplasias and anticoagulant therapy, and Dieulafoy's lesion. The real incidence of these latter lesions is difficult to assess in the context of our practice, because even when endoscopic facilities are available at the appropriate point in time, these lesions are more often than not missed, even when they have been responsible for massive UGI bleeding.

Table 9.I   Causes of Upper GI Haemorrhage in Accra

Causes	Number	Percentage (%)
DU	88	15.9
Prepyloric	36	6.5
GU	28	5.1
Lesser Curve (Type 1)	64	11.6
Gastric Erosions	2	0.4
Duodenal Erosions	7	1.3
Oesophagitis	15	2.7
Gastritis	10	1.8

Gastric Polyps	4	0.7
Duodenal Polyps	2	0.4
Oesphageal Polyps	1	0.2
Oesophageal Varices	169	30.6
Gastric Varices	4	0.7
Negative Findings	78	14.1
Total	552	100

Contd. from pg. 89:Table 9.1 Causes of Upper Gi Haemorrhage in Accra

Clinical Presentation

UGIB is announced by haematemesis (vomiting of bright red or dark blood – coffee grounds) and/or melaena (passage of black, tarry stools) or frankly bloody stools. Usually, haematemesis is generally indicative of oesophageal and gastric bleeding while melaena suggests duodenal haemorrhage; nonetheless duodenal episodes may manifest as haematemesis while gastric and oesophageal bleeding may manifest as melaena only.

Since the bleeding is usually acute and the loss significant in many cases, even in the mild cases, the presentation rapidly builds up into a resuscitation and risk assessment, even before diagnosis of presumptive origin is made.

Table 9.2   Symptoms on Presentation

Symptoms	Number	Percent (%)
Haematemesis	360	65.2
Melaena	96	17.4
Bleeding P.R.	22	4.0
Haematemesis and Melaena	31	5.6
Not indicated	43	7.8
Total	552	100.0

Initial Management

Appropriate haemodynamic assessment involves careful measurements of pulse, blood pressure, estimates of intravascular volume status, to guide resuscitation efforts. Patients with substantial intravascular loss have resting tachycardia (> 100/min) and systolic hypotension (<100 mmHg), postural hypotension, pale mucous membranes, collapsing neck veins and diminishing urinary output.[2]

The highest priority attaches to urgent volume replacement to restore haemodynamic stability. Intravenous crystalloid fluids are given through one or two wide-bore cannulae (16-18 gauge) or even central venous catheters, if peripheral access is not available.

With an eye on oxygen-carrying capacity, especially in older patients with cardiopulmonary co-morbidity, the use of supplemental oxygen, infusion of plasma expanders, and packed red cells should be encouraged.

Once a measure of cardiovascular stability has been attained, a more detailed history is taken which would establish the extent of the bleeding episode in relation to attendant symptoms referable to significant anaemia, palpitations, dizziness, fainting.

There may be previous history of dyspepsia suggestive of peptic ulcer disease, or of liver disease or of alcoholism, suggestive of oesophageal "varices". Intake of NSAIDS, asprin or recent or ongoing anticoagulation should be ascertained. Bleeding from stress ulcers may also be suggested by immediately prior major surgery or trauma, burns or fulminating sepsis or renal failure. As many of the lesser known causes of gastrointestinal bleeding should be ascertained as possible, but it is a matter of concern to the clinician that in 50 percent of patients there may be no suggestive history.

Apart from confirming the signs of significant bleeding initially noted, physical examination aims at eliciting signs referable to the two principal causes of UGIB, i.e. epigastric tenderness with or without guarding, suggestive of peptic ulcer disease and the stigmata of significant liver disease that may be responsible for oesophageal varices – hepatosplenomegaly, ascites, spider naevi and palmar erythema. Less commonly an epigastric mass indicative of a gastric carcinoma may be noted. Unusual presentations include circum oral pigmentation or telangiectasias indicating hereditary telangeactasia.

Patient Triage and Risk Stratification

The clinical diagnosis suspected from history and physical examination has to be confirmed by appropriate investigative procedure, essentially identifying the source of the bleeding to expedite treatment. Since presentation is mostly emergent it is essential that this is done expeditiously with minimal risk to the patient. Herein lies the need for patient triage and risk stratification. Urgent oesophago-gastro-duodenoscopy (OGD) has been proposed as the standard of care in patients with high risk lesions, although the precise timing of OGD has been variably defined. The American Society for Gastrointestinal Endoscopy guidelines suggest that early endoscopy within 24 hours maximizes impact on hospital length of stay, transfusion requirement, yet do not make a formal recommendation regarding optimal time for OGD within a 24 hours window[3].

However, using pre-investigative clinical variables, scoring tools have been developed to facilitate the triage or separation of bleeding patients, identifying those in need of urgent endoscopic evaluation, predicting the risk of an adverse outcome, and guiding treatment.[4] So far two risk stratification systems have been in general use: the Blatchford[5] scale ranging from 0 to 23, and the Rockall[6] scale (ranging from 0 to 11); in both systems, the higher scores indicate higher risk.

In both systems, the complete score makes use of both clinical and endoscopic criteria to predict re-bleeding or outcome. Both systems have been validated in many health settings. Unfortunately this has not been the case in the developing world, where these quantative scoring systems are not in general use. The risk stratification tends to be qualitative rather than quantitative.

The endoscopic appearance of a bleeding ulcer is often predictive of the likelihood of recurrent bleeding on basis of the Forrest classi-fication,[7] which ranges from 1A to III. High-risk lesions are charac-terized by active spurting of blood (Grade IA), oozing of blood (Grade IB), non-bleeding visible blood vessel (Grade IIA) and adherent clot, variously coloured and not readily dislodged by suction or irrigation (Grade IIB). Low-risk lesions are characteristically flat, pigmented spots (Grade IIC) with clean ulcer floor and base (Grade III).

Clearly, a multidisciplinary approach, involving a trained endoscopist with full support is the sheet anchor of management; this means 24 hours of cover ensuring that the examination is done within 24-48 hours of presentation, providing the subject is stable haemodynamically. This also improves certain outcomes – units of blood transfused, and hospital stay. Early endoscopy also allows for safe and expedited discharge of those considered as being of low risk, in the process reducing costs to the attending facilities.

High-Risk Patients

Patients so identified clinically and confirmed by endoscopic Forrest classification[7] need to be admitted to hospital and given endoscopic therapeutic management. They are therefore triaged to an intensive or high-dependency unit for monitoring in the first 24 hours, with a planned hospital care lasting about 72 hours.

Patients with active bleeding (Forrest 1A), oozing (1B), visible vessel (IIA) and adherent clot (IIB) should undergo endoscopic haemostasis; this has been shown to reduce incidence of recurrent bleeding, the need for urgent surgery, and death. An extensive arsenal of endoscopic techniques is available: injection of vasoconstricting agents (adrenaline), of saline-producing local tamponade, sclerosing agents, tissues adhesives, or thermotherapy using multiple electro-coagulation and heater probes, or non-contact methods, e.g. argon plasma coagulation, and mechanical therapy using endoscopic clips.

Endoscopic injection measures appear to supercede all other measures; nonetheless several studies[8] have shown that addition of a second haemostatic approach, e.g. contact thermal therapy further reduces the re-bleeding rates, the need for surgery and the ultimate mortality. It has been observed that the combination of vasocon-striction and volume tamponade facilitates a clear view of the bleeding vessel, permitting targeted contact thermal therapy.

For the leading workers in the field however, controversy still persists as to the superiority of combination therapy over contact thermal therapy.[9] Indeed, there is need currently, for appropriately powered clinical trials of the comprehensive range of modalities of effecting haemostasis, singly or in combination; until these are to hand, it would appear sound policy for the endoscopist to adopt the haemostatic technique he is most comfortable with, since almost all the modalities under discussion can be reasonably efficacious.

Another controversial issue is whether or not planned second-look endoscopy within 24 hours should be performed. The Society of Endoscopy has not recommended it although some recent meta-analyses have shown a significant reduction in rate of re-bleeding.[10] As a routine, a second look may not be cost-effective, but where there are clinical signs of recurrent bleeding, it is prudent not to ignore these in particular cases.

A further technical issue in need of clarification is the need for a prokinetic agent to facilitate emptying of retained blood. The American Society for Gastrointestinal Endoscopy Guidelines indicate that the use of erythromycin given i/v significantly improves mucosal visibility.[11]

Medical Therapy of Bleeding from Peptic Ulcer Patients

Pharmacotherapy over the past decade has focused on the remarkable acid suppression of proton-pump inhibitors in the treatment of patients with nonvariceal UGIB, particularly those with a peptic ulcer basis. Gastric acid has been shown[12] to impair clot formation, promote platelet disaggregation and favour fibrinolysis. Raising the gastric pH to circa 6 can be expected to promote clot stability and thus decrease the incidence of re-bleeding. No controlled trial demonstrating the efficacy of proton-pump inhibitors against H_2 blockers in this regard has been published but a pooled analysis of [16] randomized controlled trials has indicated that intravenous bolus loading followed by continuous infusion of proton-pump inhibitors is more effective in decreasing rates of re-bleeding and the need for surgery.[13]

Neoadjuvant PPI therapy prior to endoscopic haemostasis has not been demonstrated by controlled clinical trials to influence the incidence of re-bleeding, need for surgery, or the 30-day outcome. It has however become accepted practice and is indeed recommended by the international consensus guidelines[14] for pragmatic reasons, e.g. where access to prompt endoscopy or availability of the expertise is limited.

Long-Term PPI Management

After the initial therapy, patients should be given the benefit of full mucosal healing by the exhibition of triple therapy with amoxycillin, chlarythromycin and to ensure against recurrent bleeding extension of the PPI exposure for a period of 6-8 weeks. This is the more important for patients who have to continue taking NSAIDS, acetyl salicylic acid or those known to harbour *H pylori* infection.[15,16] Prolonged PPI therapy is however not without potential risks – clostridium difficile infection, community-acquired pneumonia, calcium malabsorption, resulting in osteoporosis and risk of pathological fracture. In the few patients for whom prolonged PPI is prescribed, monitoring for these signs should be implemented.

Medical therapy for bleeding peptic ulcer disease is highly efficacious; in some 10 percent of patients it may fail to respond. These include patients with a prolonged history of preceding dyspepsia, previous ulcer bleeding, presentation with shock, spurting active bleeding at endoscopy, and large ulcers (>2cm).[17] These are the indications that prompt surgical intervention. Age over 45 years is an additional factor that weighs the evidence in favour of surgical intervention. For duodenal ulcers the preferred surgical procedure is gastrotomy and suturing or under-running of the ulcers and covering of any visible vessels. Vagotomy is added in the ulcerating lesions which do not appear to match the severity of the blood loss. Gastric ulcers are similarly treated but where there are suspicions of gastric carcinoma a hemi or subtotal gastrectomy is the appropriate resectional surgery.

Interventional radiology techniques are being increasingly employed, especially in patients with uncontrolable bleeding, where endoscopic haemostatic procedures have failed, particularly where the patients are high-risk surgical candidates.

Angiographic localization of the lesion with transcatheter embolization has produced primary rates of technical success from 52 to 94 percent, with recurrent bleeding requiring repeat embolization in approximately 10 percent of patients.[18] The technical expertise required, however, limits the procedure to specialized centres.

Bleeding Oesophageal and Gastric Varices

The presentation of UGIB may be strongly suggestive of variceal origin from the large volume of blood loss causing rapid hemadynamic instability with threat of multi-organ failure. Progressive cerebral hypoxia may lead to loss of consciousness with threat of aspiration of vomitus. The stigmata of hepatobiliary disease may be evident and the large amount of blood in the GI tract would precipitate symptoms and signs of porto-systemic encephalopathy. On the other hand variceal bleeding may be less dramatic, presenting as a steady oozing manifest as persistent melaena.

The initial volume resuscitation involves blood transfusion (fresh blood), correction of coagulation abnormalities (e.g. fresh frozen plasma, platelets) making up vitamin deficiencies that may contribute to coagulation defects (e.g. Vit K, folic acid).

As variceal haemorrhage is associated with high incidence of severe bacterial infections (Gram negative septicaemia) it is expedient to carry out blood cultures and cover the patient with i/v ciprofloxacin 200mg 12-hourly and metronidazole 500 mg 6-hourly for 7 days.[19]

A number of vasoactive agents have been employed to lower portal pressure and induce splanchnic vasoconstriction and encourage temporary control of variceal haemorrhage. The leading agents include i/v vasopressin (20 units in 200 mls of 5percent dextrose over 2 hours); Glypressin, Terlipressin, Octreotide, a somatostatin analogue, (50 ugm followed by 25-50 ugm/hr for 48 hrs). These agents all have significant side effects; recent clinical trials have demonstrated preference of terlipressin over octreotide.[20] PPI infusion to counteract mucosal stress ulceration has also been shown to be beneficial.

Endoscopic Treatment of Varices

Two endoscopic procedures have been extensively utilized in the control of bleeding varices, namely (i) sclerotherapy by injecting sodium tetradeyl sulphate or ethanolamine intravariceally into collapsed veins or perivascularly, and (ii) ligation of the varices using small elastic 'O' rings. Eighty percent of varices are seen at the lower end of the oesophagus while some 20 percent occur at the cardia and fundus of the stomach. While injection sclerotherapy is readily applicable at both sites, ligation entails some technical difficulties with gastric varices, which are therefore treated mainly by injection sclerotherapy.

One major disadvantage of ligation is the need to withdraw the endoscope and re-load bands individually; newer devices have however, been developed which allow up to six-band ligations without the need for re-loading.[21]

A recent meta-analysis of studies comparing endoscopic ligation with sclerotherapy for treatment of oesaphageal variceal bleeding has concluded that ligation should be considered the endoscopic treatment of choice for patients with oesophageal varices.[22]

By whatever method is used, it is important that patients have follow-up endoscopic treatment at 2-3 weekly intervals until all varices are eradicated. Patients who prove refractory to endoscopic haemostasis face the more drastic options of balloon tamponade and surgical intervention.

Balloon Tamponade

Balloon tamponade is by consensus reserved for acute variceal bleeding which has not been controlled by endoscopic haemostatic procedure and systemic exhibition of terlipressin or octreotide.[23] The incidence of re-bleeding after removal of the balloon is however about 50 perent. Three types of tubes are in current use. The Linton-Nachlas tube has a single lumen, besides the gastric drainage tube, to be used to inflate the single fundal balloon which compresses the varices at the gastric side of the gastrooesophageal junction. The Segstaken-Blakemore tube has an oesophageal balloon as well as a gastric balloon, for both oesophageal and gastric compression.

The Minnesota tube has four lumens; two used to inflate the oesophageal and gastric balloon, while the remaining lumens allow for gastric and oesophageal aspiration; clearly the Minnesota tube is often the preferred tube for balloon tamponade. Most countries in Africa seem to stock only the Segstaken-Blakemore tube.

If control of bleeding is achieved, the oesophageal balloon is left inflated for 2 hours only, subsequently deflating the oesophageal balloon for 30-60 minutes 8 hourly. The gastric tamponade can be maintained continuously 48-72 hours, after which it is deflated and bleeding assessed before it is removed. Continued bleeding is a critical development and is an indication for surgical intervention.

Surgical Management

In principle this is undertaken through one of two modalities (i) direct attack on the varices:- oesophageal, or gastric transaction of the varices, devascularisation, endoscopic stapling or replacement through liver transplantation or (ii) methods that involve central or selective porto-systemic shunting to reduce the portal pressure.

Most of these entail major surgical procedures and should naturally be practised on patients with adequate functional hepatic reserve. The Pugh-Child classification forms the basis for selection for surgical intervention; the risk is good and acceptable with class A patients, moderate with B and poor with C.

Central Porto-systemic Shunts

Four major prospective randomized trials comparing porto caval shunting with medical therapy in cirrhotics with portal hypertension, were unanimous in their conclusion that shunting prevented re-bleeding, but worsened hepatic function, thus transforming the mode of death from exsanguination to hepatic failure.[24,25,26]

Percutaneous Shunts

A transjugular intra hepatic porto-systemic shunt (TIPS), using a balloon-expandable stent, has made the decompression of the portal vein extremely simple (Jugular vein ® inferior vena cava, ® hepatic vein ® portal vein).[27] As TIPS creates a side-to-side porto-systemic shunt, it is attended by significant porto-systemic encephalopathy (25 percent) and deterioration of liver function. The procedure is also liable to significant complications-injury to liver capsule, intra abdominal haemorrhage, infection and stent migration. Regular follow up is essential.

Selective Shunts

Selective porto-systemic shunts such as the distal spleno-renal shunt (Warren Shunt), separate the splanchnic circulation into porto-mesenteric and gastro-splenic, with the latter selectively draining blood from the oesophageal and gastric varices into the left ranal vein. As the porto-mesenteric circulation is not interfered with, portal perfusion and *ipso facto* hepatic function are largely, though not fully, maintained. The incidence of encephalopathy, though not eliminated, is much reduced.

Most prospective randomized trials to date have not shown a difference in mortality from central shunts.[28]

Less Common Causes of UGIB

Some 90 percent of Mallory – Weiss tears settle spontaneously. Where the vomiting continues and bleeding persists, endoscopic modalities should be applied though thermal coagulation should be avoided to obviate oesophageal wall perforation; band ligation is preferable.

Dieulafoy's Lesions

These lesions made up of abnormal blood vessels create diagnostic problems because they are located in the submucosa and erode the mucosa without producing an ulcer. They account for 1 percent of UGIB. The lesions are often missed when there is no active bleeding because of the absence of an ulcer. Endoscopic haemostatic measures, mainly adrenaline injection supported by thermal coagulation, are effective and safe.

Primary and Metastatic Tumours of the Upper GI Tract

These are noted to cause haemorrhage periodically. The primary neoplasms include gastric, oesophageal cancers, GI stromal tumours (GIST), lymphoma, carcinoids, Kaposi sarcoma, leiomyoma, and leiomyosarcoma. Metastatic tumours[29] from the bronchus, breast and melanoma have occasionally been reported to present with haemorrhage.

Massive haemorrhages from such tumours are not amenable for endoscopic haemostasis because the blood is mostly from tissue necrosis; resectional surgery is usually indicated.

Aorto-Enteric Fistula

The population, even in developing countries, is gradually aging, so this unusual cause for UGIB should be considered for elderly patients who complain of the triad of (i) abdominal pain (ii) palpable pulsatile epigastric mass and (iii) GI bleeding, especially when they are known to harbour aortic aneurysm or have had aortic vascular surgeries.

Endoscopy that permits visualization of the distal duodenum and proximal jejunum is essential for diagnosis and an abdominal contrast CT scan are useful in confirming the diagnosis. Treatment is invariably surgical and broad spectrum bactericidal antibiotics should be used promptly to forstal complications.

Long-Term Treatment for Post-Variceal Bleeding

Patients who are successfully treated for variceal bleeding need long-term follow up to monitor not only recurrence and further advance of variceal development but also changes in portal pressure. The mainstay for the reduction of portal pressure is the non-selective action of propranolol. It achieves this by producing splanchnic vasocon-striction and reduction of cardiac output. Starting at 40 mg bd, the dose is increased to 80 mg.[30] There is need to monitor the patient's response in view of the depressive side effects of this drug on cardiac contractility.

Conclusion

This review of UGIB has targeted common emergency presentations, but it is important for the clinician to maintain a high index of suspicion on non-emergency anaemia situations turning into an emergency, for example the persistent anaemia from unsuspected hookworm infestation that precipitates severe malaena which leads to a negative laparotomy. Patients with significant UGIB who settle spontaneously need to be investigated even more vigorously for the rarer causes that hang over these patients like the sword of Damocles. To this must be added the diagnostic problems of intermediate and lower gastrointestinal haemorrhages that masquerade as upper GI haemorrhages.

Acknowledgement

The author acknowledges the contribution of the Residents and Consultants of the Departments of Medicine and Surgery as well as the staff of the Endoscopy Centre, and also for making the mass of patient information available for study.

References

1. Stomach and.Duodenum. In: Badoe, E.A., Archampong, E.Q. and Da Rocha, AFODU (eds.), *Principles and practice of surgery including pathology in the tropics.* Accra: University of Ghana Medical School. 2009. 637-641.

2. British Society of Gastro-enterology Endoscopy Committee. Non-variceal upper gastro-intestinal haemorrhage guidelines. *Gut* 2002 51 Suppl. 4 (iv)-iv 6.

3. Adler, D. G., Leighton, J. A., Davila, R. E., Hirota, W. K., Jacobsen, B.C., Qureshi, W. A., Rajan, E., Zuckerman, M. J., Finelli, R. D., Hambrick, R. D., Baron, T., Faigel, D.O. ASGI guidelines: Role of Endoscopy in acute non-vertical upper GI haemorrhage. *Gastroenterology* 2009 23: 489-493.

4. Barkun, A., Bardou, M. and Marshall, T.K. Consensus recommendations for managing patients with non-variceal upper gastrointestinal bleeding *Ann. Intern med* 2003: 139 843-857.

5. Blatchford, D.O., Murray, W.R. and Blatchford, M. A risks core to predict need for treatment for upper-gastrointestinal haemorrhage *Lancet* 2000; 356:1318-1331.

6. Rockall, I.A., Loga, R.F., Devlins, H.B. and Northfield, T.C. Risk assessment after acute gastrointestinal haemorrhage. *Gut* 1996, 38; 316-321.

7. Forrest, J.A., Finlayson, N.D. and Sherman, D.J. Endoscopy in gastrointestinal bleeding *Lancet* 1974 2: 394-394 –7.

8.   Vergarm, M., Calvet, X. and Gisbert, J.P. Epinephrine versus epinephrine injection and a second endoscopic method in high risk bleeding ulcers. *Cochrane Database SYST.* Rev 2007, (2) CD 005584

9.   Marmo, R., Rotondano, G., Piscopo, Bianco, M.A., D'Angella R. and Cipolletta, L. Dual therapy v\sus monotherapy in endoscopic treatment of high-right bleeding ulcer: A meta-analysis of controlled trials. *Am. J. Gastroenterology* 2007:102: 279-289

10.   Marmo, R., Rotondano, G., Piscopo, R., Pisco, A. and Cipolletta L. Outcome of endoscopic treatment of peptic ulcer bleeding: is a second look necessary? A meta-analysis. *Gastrointestinal Endoscopy* 2003: 57:62-67

11.   Barkun, A.N., Bardou, M., Gralner, I.M. and Sung, J.J. Kinetics in acute upper GI bleeding: a meta analysis. *Gastrointestinal. Endoscopy* 2010; 72: 1138-1145

12.   Barkun, A.N., Cockeram, A.W., Plourde V. and Fedorak R.N. Review article acid suppression in non-variceal acute upper gastrointestinal bleeding. Aliment Pharmacol Ther. 1999 13: 1565-1584

13.   Barkun AN, Herba K, Adam V, Kennedy W, Falcone CA, Bardou M, High dose intravenous proton pomp inhibition following endoscopy therapy in the acute management of patients with bleeding peptic ulcers in the USA and Canada. A cost-effective analysis. *Aliment Pharmacol Thera.* 2004 19:591-600.

14.   Barkun, A.N., Bardou, M., Kuipers, E.J., Sung, J., Hunt, R.H., Martel, M., Sinclair, P., International consensus recommendations on management of patients with non-variceal gastrointestinal bleeding *Ann. Intern Med.* 2010: 152:101-113.

15.   Chan, F. K., Chung, S.C,, Suen, B.Y., Lee, Y.T., Leung, W. K., Leung, V.K., Wu, J.C., Lau, J.Y,, Hui, Y., Lai, M.S., Chan, H.L., Sung, J.J. Preventing recurrent upper gastrointestinal bleeding in patients with H pylori infection who are taking low dose asprin or naproxen. *New England Journal Med.* 2001 344: 967-973.

16.   Chan FK, Sung JJ, Chung SC, To KL, Nung MY, Leung VK, Lee VT, Chan CS, Li FK, Woo, J. Randomised trials of eradication of H pylori before non-steroidal anti-inflammatory drug therapy to prevent peptic ulcers. *Lancet* 1997:350: 975-979.

17.   Thomopoulos, K.C., Theocharis, G.J., Vagenas, K.A., Danikas, D.D., Vagiants, C.E., Nikolopoulou, V. N. Predictors of haemostatic failure after adrenaline injection in patients with peptic ulcers with non bleeding visible vessel. *Scand J. Gastroenterology* 2004:39:600-604.

18. Romaric, F., Loffro, Y. A., Abu, A.L., Saud Ming, D. Lin, Pramod, P. R.A.O. Recent advances in endovascular techniques for management of acute non-variceal upper gastrointestinal bleeding. *World Journal of Gastrointestinal Surgery* 2011: 3:89-100.

19. Garcia-Tsao, G. Current management of the complications of cirrhosis and portal hypertension: variceal haemorrhage, ascites and spontaneous bacterial peritonitis *Gastroenterology* 2001.120:726-748.

20. Ioannou, G., Doust. J. and Rockey, D.C. Terlepressin for acute oesophageal variceal haemorrhage *Cochrane Database Syst. Rev* 2003; CD002147.

21. Saeed, Z.A. Endoscopic oesohagogastric variceal ligation with a six-shot multiple ligation device. *American Journal Gastroenterology* 1995:90:1570.

22. Lane, L. and Cook, D. Endoscoic ligation compared with sclerotherapy for treatment of oesophageal variceal bleeding. A meta-analysis *Ann. Intern Med.* 1995 123:280-287.

23. Joffe S.N, Non-Operative management of variceal bleeding. *British Journal Surgery* 1984:71:85-9.

24. Jackson, F.C., Perrin, E.B., Felix, W.R. and Smith, A.G. A clinical analysis of the therapeutic operation *Annual Surgery* 1971:174:672-698.

25. Resakck R.H., Iber F.L., Ishihara A.M., Chalmers T.C., Zimmerman, H. A controlled study of the therapeutic porto-caval shunt. *Gastroenterology* 1974:67:843-857.

26. Raynolds, T.B., Donovan, J. A., Mikkelsen, W. P. Results of a 12 years randomized trial of porto caval shunt in patients with alcoholic liver disease and bleeding varices. *Gastroenterology* 1981:80:1005-1011.

27. Mills, P. M, Martin, P., Shaked, A., Goldstein, Colquhoun, S.D., Busutil, K.W. Tipps and liver transplantation: technical considerations. *Hepathology* 1993:18 65A.

28. Henderson, J.M. Variceal bleeding: which shunt. *Gastroenterology* 1986:91:1021- 1023.

29. De Palma, G.D., Masones, Rega M., Simeoli, I., Donisim Addeop, et al. Metastatic tumours to the stomach: clinical and endoscopic features. *World Journal of Gastroenterology* 2006:12:7326-72328.

30. John, R. and Hayes, P.C. UK guidelines on the management of variceal haemorrhage in cirrhotic patients June 2000. BSG *Guideline in Gastroenterology.*

Chapter 10
Cancer of the Colon and Rectum
S.B. Naaeder and J.C.B. Dakubo

Introduction

Population and epidemiological studies have established a marked variation in the incidence of colorectal cancer in different parts of the world. The disease is common in Western societies when compared with its incidence in developing countries in Africa, Asia and South America. The apparently low incidence of colon and rectal cancer in Africa, may be due to the enormous scourge from communicable diseases and malnutrition that had kept down life expectancy in the African as well as the lack of accurate cancer records. Colorectal cancer is a disease of older persons and therefore as a population grows older the incidence of the disease will increase on demographic grounds alone. Such increase in the average life expectancy and the incidence of colorectal cancer in some populations in Africa has been reported[1]. However, major demography- linked increases in the colorectal cancer burden in developing countries may not take place for some time because young persons will continue to form the majority of the population.

Incidence

The worldwide incidence of colorectal cancer now exceeds 1.2 million index cases per year, half of whom will die of their disease[2]. Globally, colorectal cancer is the third commonest malignant neoplasm after cancer of the lung and breast (women only). It retains its third position after lung and prostate cancer in men and rises to become the second most common cancer after breast cancer in women. It accounts for 10.0 percent of all malignant neoplasms in males and 9.4 percent of all malignant tumours in females worldwide.[2] It is slightly more common in men than in women (ratio 1.4:1).[2] The incidence is highest in Australia/New Zealand, Western Europe and North America and lowest in South America, South-Central Asia, the Middle East and Africa. Intermediate rates are noted in Eastern Europe, Latin America and parts of Asia as well as Southern Africa. Currently the incidence rates are stabilizing in Northern and Western Europe. In the USA colorectal cancer incidence has been declining in the past two decades, largely due to screening of asymptomatic individuals and removal of colorectal polyps before they progress to cancer[3]. However, the incidence of colorectal cancer is increasing in developing countries which now contribute a little over a third of new cases of colorectal cancers to the annual worldwide incidence[2]. In West Africa the incidence of colorectal is increasing, albeit, slowly. Generally, incidence rates change with time. In Ghana there has been an 8-fold increase in the number of new cases of colorectal cancer seen per year from an average of 4.1 new cases in the 1960s to an average of 32.6 new cases currently[4,5]. It is now the third most common malignant disease after cancer of the breast and liver in Ghana[6]. In Nigeria it is the fourth most common malignant neoplasm[7]. Hospital-based data in Ghana and Nigeria show the crude incidence rates of colorectal cancer to be 11.18 per 100 000 population and 3.4 per 100 000 population respectively.[5,7] These rates are far lower than the incidence rates of over 40 per 100 000 population reported in Western nations.[8]

Cancer of the colon and rectum is one of the leading causes of death from malignant disease. It is the fourth most frequent cause of cancer death worldwide accounting for 8.0 percent of cancer deaths.[2] In the USA colorectal cancer ranks third as a cause of cancer death after lung and prostate cancer in men and after lung and breast cancer in women[3]. Whereas the mortality rate from colon cancer is decreasing in the United States and Western Europe the opposite is occurring in Central and Eastern Europe and lowest in Africa.[2,8] In Ghana it is the 10th cause of cancer death overall and the 8th and 9th cause of cancer deaths in males and females respectively.[9]

Risk Factors

A number of risk factors are associated with colorectal cancer, some modifiable and others non-modifiable. The non-modifiable risk factors include age, sex and genetic factors. Cancer of the colon and rectum affects all age groups but the risk increases with age with a little over 90 percent of cases aged 50 years or older in western countries.[3] In 1960 6.7 percent of Ghanaians were 50 years or older.[10] This figure had risen to 10.0 percent by the 1990s[11] and is currently 12.1percent.[12] The number of new cases of colorectal cancer in Ghana has increased steadily over the same period in consonance with the aging population. Its highest incidence is in the seventh decade in both developed and developing countries.[1,5,13,14] Overall, colorectal cancer is slightly more common in men than in women,[1,2] however when colon and rectal cancers are considered separately colon cancer is slightly more common in women and vice versa for rectal cancer.[1]

There is general agreement that most colorectal cancers arise from sporadic adenomas: tubular, tubulo-villous and villous, which are precursor lesions for colorectal carcinoma, through the adenoma-carcinoma sequence. They usually predate the cancer by 5-15 years. The risk is higher in adenomas that are large >2cm, sessile, dysplastic and villous in nature.

Heritable conditions such as the Familial Adenomatous Polyposis Syndromes (FAP) (*Familial Adenomatous Polyposis Coli (APC), Gardener's syndrome, Turcot's syndrome, Oldfield's syndrome*) and the Hereditary Non-Polyposis Colon Cancer syndromes (HNPCC) (*Lynch syndromes I and II*) account for 5-10 percent of colorectal cancers.[15] The FAP and HNPCC are associated with mutations in the *APC* suppressor gene and DNA repair genes (*MLH1, hMSH2*) respectively. The proto-oncogenes (*K-ras, src, C-myc*) and mutations in other tumour suppressor genes(*p 53, DCC, DPC4*) and DNA repair genes (*PMS1, PMS2*) are associated with an increased risk of colorectal cancer. These together with first -degree relatives of persons with colorectal cancer or personal history of adenomatous polyps or colorectal cancer have a threefold increased risk of colorectal cancer and adenomatous polyps. Hereditary non-polypoid colon diseases such as ulcerative colitis and Crohn's disease are associated with an increased risk of colorectal cancer, the risk being higher in those with longstanding and extensive disease. Only a few cases of these heritable conditions have been seen and reported in Ghana and West Africa.[1]

The modifiable risk factors include environmental factors such as diet, changes in lifestyle, physical exercise, obesity, socio-cultural practices, tobacco and alcohol consumption. It has been estimated that differences in diet may account for 90 percent of the variations in incidence of colorectal among countries.[17] Blame has been placed upon the excessive consumption of meat and animal fat,[18] refined carbohydrates,[19] or beer[20] at the expense of fibre, fruits and vegetables.[18] In 1971, Burkitt put forward his famous hypothesis attributing dietary fibre depletion to the aetiology of colorectal cancer, based on his observation that colon cancer, adenomatous polyps, diverticular disease and appendicitis, unlike in Western countries, were uncommon in Africa.[21] Dietary fibre increases faecal bulk, dilutes the carcinogens and decreases transit time thereby diminishing the damaging effects of the carcinogens. In addition, Thornton[22] proposed that the protective role of dietary fibre was through its fermentation, by colonic bacteria, to short chain fatty acids (acetate, propionate and butyrate) which acidified the colon resulting in the inhibition of the conversion of primary bile acids to their carcinogenic secondary and tertiary derivatives. Besides, butyrate, in contrast to the other short-chain fatty acids, has been shown to suppress cell growth, to increase doubling time and to induce cell differentiation in human colon cancer cell lines.[23,24] It has therefore been postulated that the protective effect of dietary fibre against colorectal cancer may be through its fermentation to butyrate.[23] Changes in diet may not be the most important factor as recent reports in Ghana, Nigeria and elsewhere in Africa show that colorectal cancer and appendicitis are no longer uncommon diseases[5,7,25] and the victims are predominantly low-income earners who could not afford "Western-type" diets.[1,26]

Support for changes in lifestyle as a risk factor for colorectal cancer have come from migrant studies that have shown that migrants from areas of low incidence to those of high incidence generally attain rates of colorectal cancer similar to those of their host nations. Poles and Japanese who emigrated to Australia and Hawaii respectively had within one generation acquired the high incidence patterns of their new environment.[27,28] Urban residence has also been reported to be associated with an increase in risk for colorectal cancer[29]. However, urban residence in Ghana has not been accompanied by any signif-icant changes in lifestyle.[30] Other lifestyle-related risk factors for colon cancer are obesity, lack of physical exercise and excessive consumption of alcohol and cigarette smoking.

Non-neoplastic conditions associated with increased risk for colorectal cancer include radiation colitis, *Schistosoma mansoni* infestation, immunodeficiency states, biliary and genital tract diseases and ureterosigmoidostomy.

Presenting features

Most patients with colorectal carcinoma present late (6 months or more) as early symptoms are often ignored. This results in a quarter to a third of patients presenting with acute intestinal obstruction.[1,31] However, a recent study in Ghana reported a lower figure of 17.3 percent.[5] Men tend to present earlier than women. Weight loss, abdominal pain, anaemia, abdominal mass and blood or mucus per rectum are common presenting symptoms of colon cancer whilst those with rectal cancer present most commonly with rectal bleeding with passage of mucus, weight loss, anaemia and change of bowel habits (diarrhoea or constipation or alternating diarrhoea and consti-pation). In 80-90 percent of cases the tumours are palpable on digital rectal examination.[1,31,32] Many rectal tumours are ulcerated but others may be polypoid, annular or tubular. Other presenting features are borborygmi, rectal pain and tenesmus. Some may present with peritonitis from perforation or symptoms and signs of local or distant metastases such as fistulae, low back pain, hepatomegaly or ascites. Carcinoma of the colon or rectum must be distinguished from inflam-matory strictures (diverticulitis, lymphogranuloma, Crohn's disease), amoebic or schistosomal granulomata, endometriomata and the solitary ulcer syndrome.

Pathology and Dukes Classification

In Ghana and West Africa, colon cancer occurs more commonly on the right with the caecum bearing the brunt of the disease.[1,33] Similar distribution is reported in Western nations where the regular use of the flexible fibre optic sigmoidoscope, unlike in Ghana and West Africa, to remove adenomatous polyps of the left colon has ensured a proximal shift of colon cancers. In Ghana, as elsewhere, the rectum is still the most frequent site for colorectal cancer, 80 percent of which are within reach of the examining finger.[1] The majority of colorectal cancers are well differentiated (and moderately well differentiated adenocarcinomas) with about a quarter of them being undifferentiated.

Colorectal cancers spread circumferencially more commonly than longitudinally, the latter mode of spread being limited to 1-2cm distally except in anaplastic tumours.[31] Transmural spread may lead to invasion of local structures such as the mesorectum, prostate, seminal vesicles, bladder, vagina and uterus. Lymphatic spread tends to be upwards to the draining lymph nodes and blood borne metastases go to the liver, lung, bone, brain and adrenals. Approximately 30 percent of patients have occult liver metastases at the time of presentation.[34] Transperitoneal spread to the visceral and parietal as well as the pelvic peritoneum and ovaries may give rise to ascites, Blummer's shelf on rectal examination and Krukenburg's tumours respectively.

Dukes stage A tumours are infrequently diagnosed, reportedly varying in frequency from 4-6 percent through 15 percent to 25 percent.[1,35,36,37] The US Surveillance, Epidemiology and End Results (SEER) 2008 report showed that 13.7 percent of colorectal cancers at presentation were Dukes A, 27.9 percent Dukes B, 37.2 percent Dukes C and 21.2 percent Dukes 'D'.[38] In Ghana, as elsewhere, the majority of patients with colorectal cancer present late and therefore have higher Dukes stages of the disease (Dukes B_2, C_1, C_2 and 'D')[1,5]. Screening studies have shown that twice as many tumours (70-80%) confined to the bowel wall (Dukes stages A and B) are diagnosed in screened populations as against 30-40 percent in control groups.[39,40] The absence of population screening programmes in African and other developing countries, therefore, accounts for the low incidence of early stage disease in publications emanating from these parts of the world.

Investigations

The diagnosis of colorectal carcinoma and its extent may be confirmed by diagnostic and staging investigations. Rigid proctosigmoidoscopy and flexible sigmoidoscopy both have sensitivities of 85 percent and the colonoscope, which is designed to reach the caecum and capable of detecting all neoplasms, has a sensitivity of 95 percent.[41] Figure 10.1 shows an endoscopic view of low rectal carcinoma. Biopsies, for histological confirmation, are done. Double-contrast barium enema is the investigation of choice in resource-limited areas and where colonoscopy is incomplete or impossible. It has a sensitivity of 85 percent and can demonstrate 92 percent of tumours of the colorectum.[41] CT colonography, also known as virtual colonoscopy or CT pneumocolon, is the latest addition to the armamentarium for investigating colorectal diseases. It is superior to conventional barium enema examinations. The extent of the disease is assessed with ultrasonography, abdominal and/or endoluminal, abdominal CT scanning, MRI scanning and intravenous urogragphy. Baseline carcinoembryonic antigen (CEA) levels will be useful in subsequent follow up. Supportive haematological and biochemical investigations as well as electrocardiography, chest radiography and urinalysis are essential.

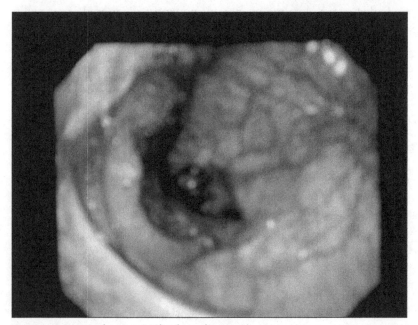

Figure 10.1: Low rectal cancer visualized at endoscopy

Treatment

For many years surgical excision has been the linchpin of treatment of colorectal cancer and it still remains so today. However, over 90 percent of tumours are detected when transmural spread has already occurred and surgery is unlikely to result in cure[14]. Despite this dismal picture surgery still offers the only hope of cure for approximately half of the victims.[14,42] In Ghana and West Africa resection rates are low, 60-75 percent for colon cancers and 43-45 percent for rectal cancer.[1,5,32,33] This is in contrast to those of western nations.[43] Nearly a third of patients with rectal cancer in our sub-region refuse surgery on account of the social unacceptability of a stoma and its attendant psychological problems.[33] Locally, 'curative' resection was possible in 60 percent and 83 percent respectively of those who underwent resection for colon and rectal cancer[1].

The early optimism that greeted adjuvant therapy in colorectal cancer has not been sustained due to the lack of significant improvements in survival following these modalities of treatment. However, chemoradiation has been and still is the standard of care for rectal tumours staged beyond Dukes Stage B1. Pre-operative and post-operative radiotherapy for rectal cancer has demonstrated marginal improvements in disease-free survival and overall survival.[31] Recent studies of preoperative chemoradiation using 5-fluorouracil/radiotherapy and 5-fluorouracil/irinothecan/radiotherapy combinations have shown some improvements in pathologic complete response rates following resection of distal rectal cancer.[44]

The most frequently used cytotoxic agent is 5-Fluorouracil in combination with leucovorin. Adjuvant cytotoxic chemotherapy in colorectal cancer has been assessed extensively in randomized control trials but the survival benefits remain small. The QUASAR trail involving 3,238 patients with colorectal cancer showed a survival benefit of only 1-5 percent.[45] A meta-analysis of randomized trials involving 3,182 patients also showed a survival benefit of up to 5.7 percent[46]. Newer agents, capecitabine, irinothecan and oxaliplatin, have recently been introduced for the treatment of metastatic disease with moderate outcomes.[31] Experience with adjuvant therapy –

radiotherapy, chemotherapy and immunotherapy – in Ghana and the sub-region is limited.

Recent advances in immunotherapy has seen a move away from the use of non-specific immunomodulators, such as lavamisole, to more targeted therapies. Three monoclonal antibodies have so far been recommended for the treatment of metastatic colorectal cancer. They include bevacizumab (Avastin) which is an anti-angiogenetic factor to tumour vascular growth, cetuximab (Erbitux) and panitumumab (Vectibix) that inhibit the effects of hormone-like factors that promote cancer growth. The limitation to general use of these monoclonal antibodies is their high cost.

Primary inoperable colorectal cancer and local recurrent disease following treatment still present management challenges to caregivers. With the introduction of thermal ablation techniques, radiofrequency electric current and more recently microwave ablation, patients with inoperable and local recurrent colorectal cancer may have some hope as early results are encouraging.[47]

Prognosis

Despite increased awareness of colorectal cancer, development of sensitive diagnostic techniques, improvements in surgical techniques and extent of resection half the patients with colorectal cancer still die of their disease within 5 years worldwide.[2] It is the second most common cause of cancer death after lung cancer in men and breast cancer in women in western nations. Factors affecting prognosis include the stage of the disease, age, obstruction or perforation, histological grade and lypmhovascular invasion. In western nations 5-year survival figures for Dukes stage A, B_1, B_2, C, and 'D' are 100 percent, 90 percent, 70 percent and 40 percent respectively. In Ghana and West Africa and indeed in Sub-Saharan Africa post-treatment follow up is poor and therefore long term survival data are not available.[1,5,32,33]

Screening

Survival from colorectal cancer depends on the stage of the disease at the time of diagnosis. To reduce the 50 percent mortality associated with colorectal cancer, the disease must be detected in its early stage when it is potentially curable. In the past four decades there has been a move towards screening of asymptomatic individuals in an attempt to detect early neoplasms in order to interrupt or delay the natural course of the disease. In developed countries, case-control studies have shown a 60-70 percent reduction in the risk of death from colorectal cancer in screened populations as compared to controls.[48] In developing countries including Ghana, screening programmes are not available and colorectal cancer will continue to be diagnosed when mural or transmural spread has already occurred. A reduction in worldwide mortality from colorectal cancer is, therefore, unlikely to be attained for many more years to come.

References

1. Naaeder, S.B. and Archampong, E.Q. Cancer of the colon and rectum in Ghana: a 5-year prospective study. *Br. J. Surg.* 1994; 81: 456-459.

2. GLOBOCAN 2008. Cancer Fact Sheet. Colorectal cancer incidence and mortality worldwide in 2008. Summary. IARC 2010.

3. American Cancer Society. Cancer Facts and Figures 2012. Atlanta, Ga. American Cancer Society 2012.

4. Badoe, E.A. Malignant disease of the gastrointestinal tract in Korle Bu Hospital, Accra, Ghana. 1956-1965. *West Afr. J. Med.* 1966; 15: 181-185.

5. Dakubo, J.C.B., Naaeder, S.B., Tettey, Y. and Gyasi, R.K. Colorectal carcinoma: An update of current trends in Accra. *West Afr. J. Med.* 2010; 29: 178-183.

6. Biritwum, R.B., Gulaid, J. and Amaning, A.O. Pattern of diseases or conditions leading to hospitalization at Korle Bu Teaching Hospital, Ghana in 1996. *Ghana medical Journal.* 2000; 34: 197-205.

7. Irabor, D.O., Arowolo, A. and Afolabi, A.A. Colon and rectal cancer in Ibadan, Nigeria: An update. *Colorectal Disease* 2010; 12: e43-e49.

8. Haggar, F.A. and Boushey, R.P. Colorectal cancer epidemiology: incidence,mortality,survival and risk factors. *Clin. Colon Rectal Surg.* 2009; 22: 191-197.

9. Wiredu, E.K. and Armah, H.B. Cancer mortality patterns in Ghana: a 10-year review of autopsies and hospital mortality. *BMC Public Health* 2006; 6: 159. http://www.biomedcentral.com/147-2458/6/159.

10.   Population Censuses Office, Population Census 1960. Accra: GPC, 1960.

11.   Population Censuses Office. Population Census 1984. Accra: GPC, 1984.

12.   Ghana Stastistical Service. 2010 Population and Housing Census. Summary Report of Final Results. May, 2012. Accra:GSS.

13.   Office of Population Censuses and Surveys. Cancer Statistics. Registration 1986. England and Wales. Series MB1. No. 19 London: HMSO 1991.

14.   McArdle, C. S., Hole,D., Hansell, D., Blumgart, L. H., Woods, C.B. Prospective study of colorectal cancer in the West of Scotland: 10-year follow-up. *Br. J. Surg.* 1990; 77: 280-2.

15.   Jackson-Thompson, J. et al. Descriptive epidemiology of colorectal cancer in the United States, 1998-2001. *Cancer.* 2006; 105(5, suppl): 1103-1111. [PubMed].

16.   Nkrumah, K.N. Inflammatory bowel disease at Korle Bu Teaching Hospital: Case reports. *Ghana Medical Journal.* 2000; 34: 32-35.

17.   Doll, R. and Peto, R. The causes of: Quantitative estimates of avoidable risks of cancer in the United States today. J. Natl. *Cancer Inst.* 1981; 66: 1191-1308.

18.   Giovannucci, E., Stampfer, M. J., Colditz, G., Rimm, E.B., and Willet, W.C. Relationship of diet to risk of colorectal adenoma in men. *J Natl Cancer Inst* 1992; 84: 91-8.

19.   Bristol, J.B., Emmett, P.M., Heaton, K.W. and Williamson, R.C.N. Sugar, fat and the risk of colorectal cancer. *Brit. Med. J.* 1985, 291: 1467-1470.

20.   McMichael, A.J., Potter, A.J. and Hetzel, B.S. Time trends in colorectal cancer mortality in relation to food and alcohol consumption: United States, United Kingdom, Australia and New Zealand. *Int. J. Epidemiol.* 1979; 8: 295.

21.   Burkitt, D.P. Epidemiology of cancer of the colon and rectum. *Cancer* 1971; 28: 3-13.

22.   Thornton, J.R. High colonic pH promotes colorectal cancer. *Lancet* 1981; i: 1081-2.

23.   Whitehead, R.H., Young. G.P. and Bhathal, P. S. Effect of short chain fatty acids on new human colon carcinoma cell line (LIM 1215). *Gut* 1986; 27: 1457-63.24.   Leavitt, J., Barrett, J.C., Crawford, B.D. and Tsao, P.O.P. Butyric acid suppression of the in vitro neoplastic state of Syrian hamster cells. *Nature* 1978; 271: 262-5.

25.   Clegg-Lamptey, J.N.A. and Naaeder, S.B. Appendicitis in Accra: A contemporary appraisal. *Ghana Medical Journal* 2003; 37: 52-56.

26.   Naaeder, S.B. and Archampong, E.Q. Acute appendicitis and dietary fibre intake. *West Afr. J. Med.* 1998; 17: 264-7.

27.   Staszewski, J., McCall. M.G. and Stenhouse, N.S. Cancer mortality in 1962-66 among Polish migrants to Australia. *Br. J. Cancer* 1971; 25: 599-610.

28.   Haenszel, W. and Kurihara, M. Studies of Japanese migrants. I. Mortality from cancer and other diseases among Japanese in the United States. *J. Natl. Cancer Ints.* 1968; 40: 43-68.

29.   Boyle, P. and Langman, J. S. ABC of colorectal cancer: Epidemiology. *Br. Med. J.* 2000; 321: 805- 808.

30.   Opare-Obisaw, C., Fianu, D.A.G. and Awadzi, K. Changes in family food habits: the role of migration. *J. Consumer Studies and Home Economics* 2008; 24: 145-9.

31.   Russell, R.C.G., Williams, N.S. and Bulstrode, CJ.K., eds. *Bailey & Love's Short Practice of Surgery.* London: Hodder Arnold, 2004: 1219-1241.

32.   Adekunle, O.O. and Lawani, J. A. Clinical aspects and management of carcinoma of the rectum in Nigerians. *East Afr. Med. J.* 1982; 59: 206-213.

33.   Adekunle, O.O. and Abioye, A. A. Adenocarcionma of the large bowel in Nigerians: A clinicopathologic study. *Dis. Col. & Rectum* 1980; 23: 559-563.

34.   Finlay, I.G., Meek D.R., Gray H.W., et al. Incidence and detection of occult hepatic metastases in colorectal carcinoma. *Br. Med. J.* 1982; 284: 803-5.

35.   Stower, M.J. and Hardcastle, J.D. The results of 1115 patients with colorectal cancer treated over an 8-year period in a single hospital. *Eur. J. Surg. Oncol.* 1985; 11: 119-23.

36.   Vellacott, K.D., Smith, J.H.F. and Mortensen, N. J. McC. Rising detection rate of symptomatic Duke's A colorectal cancers. *Br. J. Surg.* 1987; 74: 18-20.

37.   Jarvinen, H.J., Ovaska, J. and Mecklin, J. P. Improvements in the treatment and prognosis of colorectal carcinoma. *Br. J. Surg.* 1988; 75: 25-27.

38.   Reis, L.A.G., Melbert D., Krapcho, M., Strinhcomb, D.G., Howlader, N., Horner M.J.et al. (eds.). SEER Cancer Statistics Review, 1975-2005, National Cancer Institute, MD. http// seer.cancer.gov/csr/1975-2005/,

based on November 2007 SEER data submission, posted to the SEER website, 2008.

39. Winawer, S.J., Schottenfeld, D. and Flehinger, B. J. Review of colorectal cancer screening. *J. Natl. Cancer Inst.* 1991; 83: 243-53.

40. Hardcastle, J.D., Thomas W.M., Chamberlain J. et al. Randomised controlled trial of faecal occult blood screening for colorectal cancer: the results of the first 107,349 subjects. *Lancet* 1989; i: 1160-4.

41. Eddy, D.M. Screening for colorectal cancer. *Ann. Int. Med.* 1990; 88: 820-37.

42. Greenwald, P. Colon cancer overview. *Cancer* 1992; 70: 1206-1215.

43. Kingston, R.D.,Walsh, S. and Jeacock, J. Colorectal surgeons in district general hospitals produce similar survival outcomes to their teaching hospital colleagues: review of 5-year survivals in Manchester. *J. R. Coll. Surg. Edinb.* 1992; 37: 235-7.

44. Mitchell, E.P., Winter, K., Mohiuddin M. et al. Randomized phase II trial of pre-operative combined modality chemoradiation for distal rectal cancer. *Journal of Clinical Oncology* 2004; 22 (14S) July 15 Supplement: 3535.

45. Gray, R.G., Barnwell, J. and Hills, R. et al. QUASAR: A randomized study of adjuvant chemotherapy (CT) vs observation including 3228 colorectal cancer patients. *Journal of Clinical Oncology* 2004; 22 (14S) July 15 Supplement: 3501.

46. Buyse, M., Zeleniuch-Jacquotte, A. and Chalmers, T.C. Adjuvant therapy of colorectal cancer – Why we still don't know. *JAMA* 1988; 259: 3571-8.

47. Ripley, R.I., Gajdos C., Reppert A.E. et al. Sequential radiofrequency ablation and surgical debulking for unresectable colorectal carcinoma: Thermo-surgical ablation. *Journal of Surgical Oncology* 2012; Wiley Periodicals, Inc. 1-4.

48. Selby, J.V., Friedman, G.D., Quesenberry, C.P. and Weiss, N.S. . A case-control study of screening sigmoidoscopy and mortality from colorectal cancer. *N. Engl. J. Med.* 1992; 326: 658-62.

49. Ghana Statistical Service. 2000 *population and housing census. Summary report pf. final results* March 2002.

50. Badoe, E.A. Malignant tumours of the large bowel (including rectum) Korle Bu Hospital Accra, 1970-75. *Ghana Medical Journal* 1977; 16: 157-159.

Chapter 11
Lower Gastrointestinal Bleeding
E. Q. Archampong

Introduction

Historically two categories of gastrointestinal bleeding have been recognized, namely "upper" and "lower", in relation to origins proximal and distal respectively to the ligament of Treitz. However, recent advances in endoscopic procedures, in particular increasing use of capsule endoscopy, have prompted a rethinking of this classification with a proposal for "upper" "mid" and "lower" categories".[1,2]

In this system, upper GI Bleeding (UGIB) is recognised as occurring proximal to the ampulla of Vater, within reach of the oesophago-gastro-duodenoscope; mid-GI bleeding (MGIB) is defined as occurring between the ampulla and the terminal ileum, best assessed by capsule endoscopy or double balloon endoscopy (DBE), while lower GI bleeding (LGIB) is newly recognized as occurring within the colon and best evaluated by colonoscopy.

In most parts of the world, mid and lower source of bleeding account for 25-30 percent of all GI bleeding.[3,4] In developing countries the presentation may be chronic, as longstanding anaemia, but many also present acutely with much haemodynamic instability[5,6] demanding urgent resuscitation and management. Although the more sophisticated investigative procedures are not consistently available in developing countries, it is important that whenever possible the new concept of classification be used in patient management. This article reviews recent experience of mid and lower GI bleeding at our centre, with emphasis on initial evaluation, diagnostic procedures and definitive management.

Materials and Methods

For this review the records of 675 patients who were referred from the surgical and medical outpatients and general services to the

Endoscopy Unit from October 2010 to end of September 2012 were analysed retrospectively. The aetiological distribution of these patients and the symptoms they presented with are depicted in Tables 11.1 and 11.2. Clearly the vast majority of patients complaining of rectal bleeding had haemorrhoids but it is significant that 7.0 percent had colorectal cancer.

Nearly 6 percent had significant bleeding from diverticular disease and only a few (1.9 percent) suffered from fissure in ano. Clearly vascular lesions such as angiodysplasias are difficult to identify; only 3 were diagnosed in the two years reviewed. It is note worthy that 2.2 percent of undiagnosed iron deficiency anaemias were traceable to colorectal lesions.

Patients with negative findings were separately documented. The demographic and epidemiological distribution of patients seen at the Endoscopy Unit is currently uncertain; it is certainly not representative of the population in the Greater Accra Region. The incidence figures arrived at in this study are therefore only approximations of the true position in the population as a whole.

Table 11.1 **Aetiological Factors in LGIB**

FACTOR	NUMBER	%
Haemorrhoids	474	70.2
Diverticular Disease	40	5.9
Colorectal Carcinoma	47	7.0
Polyps (Single) (Multiple)	30 35 5	5.2
Colitis (Practitis)	14 13	2.0 1.9
Angiodysplasia	3	0.4
Granuloma (Amoebic)	2	0.3
Normal mucosa	47	7.0
Total	675	100.0

Table 11.2 Symptomatology in LGIB

	NUMBER	%
Bleeding P.R.	547	18.1
LGIB	91	13.5
Melaena	9	1.3
Anaemia (Occuit Blood)	15	2.2
Not Recroded	13	1.9
Total	675	100

Initial Management and Resuscitation

Some 80 percent of patients with acute mid and lower GI bleeding experience spontaneous cessation of bleeding within 24 hours of admission. Patients with continued bleeding—as occurs in diverticular disease, inflammatory diseases or amoebiasis—may however rapidly deteriorate and present in a haemodynamically unstable state, demanding urgent diagnosis and treatment. The principles involving implementation of "ABC" apply, securing the airway and obtaining adequate venous access for appropriate volume resuscitation. The attainment of a reasonable clinical stability is the signal for a thorough history focusing on intake of anticoagulants and antiplatelet agents, and physical examination that would lead on to the diagnosis. Appropriate laboratory tests, in particular haemoglobin, haematocrit grouping and cross matching, and coagulation profile, are conducted. Where haemorrhagic shock threatens on account of continued active bleeding, resuscitation and evaluation are carried out concurrently.

In these severely ill patients, especially in the elderly, it is crucial to apply the principles of "damage control" resuscitation, ensuring early exhibition of blood and blood products, and oxygen therapy to help to correct the lethal triad of coagulopathy, metabolic acidosis and hypothermia, and thus influence the outcome is crucial.[7]

Diagnosis, Localisation, and Interventional Therapies

It has been established that in any situation that presents as lower GI bleeding, the source may indeed lie in the upper tract in some 12 percent of cases.[8] Localisation should therefore begin with passing an NG tube.

The finding of blood in the tube would suggest, but is not pathognomonic of, an upper GI bleed. Oesophago-gastro-duodenoscopy (OGD) is then called for to localize such UGIB. On the other hand, the finding of bile only in the aspirate may eliminate an UGIB, though it should not entirely discount further evaluation by OGD.

With an UGIB source virtually eliminated, and providing that the patient is haemodynamically stable, urgent colonoscopy has been strongly advocated as the initial investigation of choice for localizing acute lower GIB (Figure 11.1). Colonoscopy has high diagnostic accuracy and capacity for therapeutic intervention even in the unprepared colon[9,10,] Lhewa and Strate[11] report diagnostic accuracy of 74-100 per cent with standard colonic preparation. This compares with an accuracy of 40-70 percent with the radionuclide scanning diagnostic modality.[12] Angiography is even less sensitive on account of the need for higher rates of bleeding. Colonoscopy also has the advantage that a number of techniques – injection of adrenaline, thermal coagulation as well as clips and band ligation— may be used for endoscopic haemostasis once the source of bleedings is identified.[11] Furthermore, in terms of safety (low complication rates) and improved outcomes such as low re-bleeding rates and the need for surgery, colonoscopy is currently the preferred mode of investigation and localization. There is need, however, for larger randomized trial to define its efficacy.

There are a number of draw backs associated with colonoscopy: - the need for bowel preparation especially in urgent actively bleeding patients; the need for sedation and assistance by experienced staff; the low prevalence of stigmata of colonic haemorrhage and difficulty in predicting recurrence of bleeding. These are challenges that have to be addressed in the application of what is currently the preferred modality for confirmation of diagnosis and localization of LGIB.

Where colonoscopy confirms the presence of blood in the colon, but cannot accurately localize the source of bleeding, radiographic modalities, if available, may solve the problem. Interventional angiography can detect bleeding at rates above 0.5ml/min and offers the potential for trans-catheter embolisation as a means of controlling the haemorrhage. Unfortunately, these modalities are as yet not available in many developing countries. In their absence many patients have no option but to be optimized for the more sever alternative of surgical intervention.

Radionuclide scanning is sensitive and able to detect bleeding rates as low as 0.1ml/min.[13] Indeed, it is able to detect slower rates of bleeding than angiography, but the limiting factors here are that the procedure localizes active bleeding to a region of the abdomen, rather than a specific luminal anatomical site, and therapeutic intervention is not practicable.

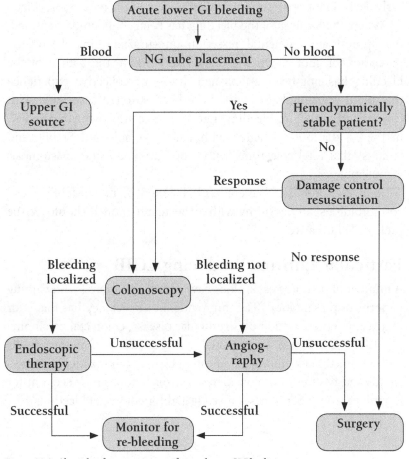

Figure 11.1: Algorithm for management of acute lower GI Bleeding

Surgical Intervention

Most patients with LGIB settle spontaneously and may not come to a consideration for surgical intervention. The indications for acute surgery include massive bleeding with haemodynamic instability and recurrent bleeding. The surgery tends to involve major resections. Unfortunately the prospective candidates tend to be elderly, with multiple co-morbidities, for whom such surgery would appear "aggressive". This category of patient also happens to be the group least receptive to the repetitive physiological interventions that characterize normal operative therapy. Paradoxically therefore, for this group, an early decision for brisk surgical intention may be the most appropriate.

Where the location of the bleeding has been confidently identified, the appropriate segmental resection on surgical principles is the procedure of choice. On the other hand, where the source of the bleeding has not been established, it is our collective experience that blind segmental resections have been so often associated with unacceptably high re-bleeding rates and accompanying morbidity; in these situations we agree with Farner et al.[14] and Stabile and Stamos[15] that total colectomy with a primary ileo-rectal anastomosis is preferable.

In a compromised patient with haemodynamic instability and co-morbidities, an ileostomy with a Hartmann's pouch should be the preferred alternative.

Particular Entities Producing LGIB

A number of pathological entities have been encountered with varying patterns of presentation. The improving life expectancy has made for increasing representation of diverticular disease, colorectal carcinoma and to a lesser degree inflammatory disease such as ulcerative colitis and Crohn's disease among the causes of LGIB in our practice. Haemorrhoids and fissures once considered unusual entities now account for a significant number of cases investigated for colorectal bleeding.

Diverticular Disease

Formerly considered uncommon in surgical practice in developing countries, diverticular disease is increasingly being encountered in recent years,[5,16] frequently with complications, usually bleeding or diverticulitis with perforation. Though 90 percent of diverticula occur in the left colon, bleeding episodes take place in the right colon at least 50 percent of the time.[17]

Colonic diverticula are pulsion diverticula or out-pouchings of the mucosa and submucosa of the colon, often associated with situations of increased intra-luminal pressure within the colon. These often occur along lines of weakness occupied by connective tissue septa between the bundles of the circular muscle coat; it is through these septa also that the intra-luminal branches of the marginal artery of the colon penetrate the colonic wall from serosa to submucosa. This artery is intimately related to the neck and fundus of the diverticulum, being separated from its lumen by only mucosa and a few strands of attenuated muscle fibres. Injurious factors e.g. mechanical agents from faecoliths or systemic hypertension, induce eccentric intimal thickening and scarring of the associated *vasa recta,* predispose to rupture and massive bleeding, which is more often intra-luminal than into the serosal or pericolic tissues.

Characteristically there is no inflammatory process, acute or chronic, around the diverticular bleeding, so diverticulitis is not a precipitating agent in the cause of the bleeding.

Hypertension, however, is a predisposing factor; so also are antico-agulation, diabetes mellitus and ischaemic heart disease.

In terms of clinical diagnosis, bleeding is infrequent, occurring in 3 to 5 percent of patients with diverticulosis, but it is the most common cause of life-threatening lower GI haemorrhage in diverticular disease. It is sudden and ceases spontaneously in 90 percent of cases. Longsteth[18] has predicted the recurrence rate over time at 9 percent in 1 year, 10 percent at 2 years, 90 percent at 3 years and 25 percent at 4 years, and this pattern should influence treatment.

Since 90 percent of patients cease bleeding spontaneously it is evident that the approach to treatment should be conservative. Jensen[19] has shown that if the bleeding lesion is spotted endoscopically, haemostosis through this technique has a good chance of success with very low rates of recurrent bleeding. Bakhari et al. have reported equally good outcomes over years with just close follow up.[20]

Our experience at Korle Bu endorses this observation. Where endoscopy fails to locate the cause and source of bleeding, angiography is the next logical procedure if it is available. This may be combined with selective infusion of vasopressin and/or selective embolisation. Variable success rates have been claimed with attendant complications and recurrence rates of 15 to 20 percent.[21]

Exploratory surgical intervention is indicated in patients with ongoing recurrent bleeding if endoscopic haemostasis or angiography are not available. Patients with one recurrence certainly deserve serious consideration for resection since the risk of further episodes increases with time. Other doctors have placed emphasis on waiting for the third episode[22]; this may not be practicable. There is need to individualize the decision process, paying particular attention to attendant circumstances such as age – advancing age and co-morbidities; these are factors that urge earlier surgical intervention.

Surgery may indeed be urgent in some cases, but it is essential to have the site of bleeding in mind before laparotomy; this limits the length of colonic resection and also helps to avoid blind segmental resections, now known to be associated with significant re-bleeding rates and increased morbidity and mortality, which may rise up to 25 percent.[23] At surgery, a practical procedure that has often worked at our centre is the isolation of segments of suspicious bowel using soft intestinal clamps, and watching for the filling up of the segments with the continuing bleeding. Admittedly, this may on occasion not work. In such situations there is no alternative to total colectomy with ileo-rectal anastomosis.

Haemorrhoids

These are common, affecting 4-10 percent of the general population and accounting for up to 14 percent of cases of haematochezia. Worldwide they are the most common cause of lower GI bleeding in patients under the age of 50.[24] For many years haemorrhoids were considered rare in developing countries, especially in the tropics.

Clearly this notion must be attributed to the low level of information and investigation into the health problems of the developing world. As in the rest of the world, haemorrhoids are indeed very common in West Africa and in our series far exceeds frequency in the developed world as cause for rectal bleeding.

The classic presentation - painless passage of fresh blood, usually preceeding the stool or sometimes after the bulk of the stool, "the splash in the pan", facilitates the diagnosis. It is less often recognized that haemorrhoidal bleeding, because of the repetitive loss of small amounts of blood over a protracted time, is a most potent cause for chronic iron deficiency anaemia in both male and female adults, who may present with profound anaemia down to levels of Hb 1-2 G/dl. It is essential that even cases that present in the classic fashion are all adequately investigated since significant predisposing pathology is often discovered requiring urgent attention, e.g. associated rectal carcinoma, which may have precipitated the haemorrhoids.

The management of haemorrhoids is based on the stage of the disease at presentation. Adequate fluid and fibre intake is the primary treatment for symptomatic haemorrhoids, buttressed by change in lifestyle that ensures regular physical exercise. Bleeding first-degree haemorrhoids respond to courses of sclerotherapy, band ligation, or simple manipulations such as haemorrhoidopexy or infra-red coagulation, bicap coagulation and cryotherapy. Bulky third-degree haemorrhoids are best dealt with by the newer, less distressing procedures used in haemorrhoidectomy.

Colorectal Cancer and Polyps

Though less commonly encountered than in the Western world, an increasing number of patients with colorectal cancer are presenting with lower GI bleeding. Worldwide some 19 percent of cases of lower GI bleeding are attributed to colorectal carcinoma and polyps;[25] this is significantly different from the figure of 7.0 percent encountered in our series. The bleeding episode usually expedites diagnosis of the underlying colorectal cancer. Management follows essentially standard therapeutic principles and the outcome of treatment has not been demonstrated to be different from the other patterns of presentation of colorectal cancer.

Inflammatory Bowel Disease

Inflammatory bowel disease, consisting mainly of Crohn's disease and ulcerative colitis, is not frequently encountered as a disease entity in developing countries. In recent years rectal bleeding as a presentation for ulcerative colitis is beginning to assume importance in Ghana.[26] The establishment of the diagnosis presents a challenge and entails repeated tissue sampling through endoscopic examinations and serological tests. Management follows the usual procedures in the regular forms of presentation of inflammatory bowel disease. The differential diagnosis involves other granulomatous diseases of the colon and rectum that may present with bleeding, namely, amoebic colitis and granulomas, tuberculosis, schistosomiasis and *lympho granuloma venerium.*

Diagnosis supported by tissue studies, leads to successful systemic antibiotic and other chemotherapeutic measures.

Obscure GIB

This is the ultimate challenge in the management of gastro-intestinal bleeding; by definition this is bleeding that persists or recurs without obvious aetiology after oesophago-gastroduenescopy, colonoscopy and radiological evaluation of the small bowel, and could be catego-rised into obscure overt or obscure occult bleeding on the basis of presence or absence of clinically evident bleeding.[27]

Occult bleeding is detected by the facecal occult blood test and has seldom been studied beyond the context of colorectal cancer screening. Indeed it is considered accepted practice not to recommend further diagnostic work up, if the test result is positive and the indicated colon cancer screening work up are negative, in the absence of iron deficiency anaemia and gastrointestinal symptoms.

Obscure GI bleeding could be due to lesions that are overlooked in the oesophagus, stomach, duodenum and colon for various reasons and circumstances, in the initial work up, or lesions in the small bowel that are difficult to visualize with conventional endoscopy with radiological imaging or scintiscanning. The recent arrival of capsule endoscopy and Double Balloon endoscopy (DME) has enormously enhanced the diagnostic capacity in small bowel disease. Approximately 5 percent of patients presenting with GI haemorrhage have no source found at upper endoscopy or colonoscopy. In some 75 percent of these patients the lesion is detected in the small bowel. In those with overt bleeding (melaena, haematochezia) small bowel angiectasias are detected in 30-60 percent of the examinations.[28] It is also of interest that GI angiectasias are often associated with quantitative and/or qualitative defects in the platelet glycoprotein, called the von Willebrand's factor, resulting in the systemic bleeding disorder, von Willebrands disease.[29]

Importance of history and physical examination cannot be overemphasized in evaluation of the patient with obscure GI bleeding. The persistence and recurrent nature of the haematemesis, severity and temporal pattern of the anaemia reflected in slow decline of the haematochrit are noteworthy. A detailed history of consumption of over-the-counter medications is very important in order to exclude medication-related mucosal lesions that may exacerbate bleeding.

Skin lesions--vascular-- entities on the lips, nasal mucosa, tongue, palms, palate, nail beds, soles of feet and even the tympanic membrane-- may point to intestinal telangiectasia. Other forms of cutaneous stigmata – *dermatitis herpetiformis*, Henoch-Scho-enlein purpura may be associated with severe GI bleeding.

Apart from repeat standard endoscopy targeting rarities such as Dieulafoy's and Cameron's lesions, investigations concentrating on the small intestine have to be initiated. The outstanding procedures here are capsule endoscopy and double balloon endoscopy. The International Conference on Capsule Endoscopy Statement 2005,[115] endorsed capsule endoscopy as currently the preferred test, or mucosal imaging of the entire intestine, and should be the initial investigation in patients with obscure GIB. The only drawback is the lack of any means of non-operative interventional haemostasis; it is difficult to avoid intra-operative enteroscopy.

In the final analysis, the extent of the evaluation of the patient with obscure GIB is dependent on two major factors; the extent of the bleeding and the age of the patient. Patients with positive occult result blood test in the stool and unsustained sustained anaemia do not require further evaluation beyond periodic colonoscopy in the absence of continuing GI symptoms. Patients with ongoing transfusion requirements need full evaluation. Those over 60 years of age are most likely to be bleeding from angiectasias in up to 80 per cent of cases. Small bowel tumours are the most likely cause in those younger than 50 years of age and may be treated laparoscopically or by open laparotomy. Decision making in the older age group is more difficult because the natural history of these angiectasias is yet to be worked out.

It is estimated that less than 10 percent of such patients actually bleed and the behaviour once bleeding occurs is also uncertain although it is presumed that as many as 50 percent may never bleed. In this situation, watchful waiting with an eye on frequency of bleeding episodes and decline in the haematocrit level may determine the need for surgical intervention.

Conclusion

LGIB is not only less frequently encountered but also presents a less dramatic picture than upper GIB. There is a wide range of aetiological factors, from the common haemorrhoids and anal fissures to the rare angiodysplasias of the colon. There is also the problem of the obscure LGIB of uncertain aetiology that persists after negative oesophago-gastro-duodenoscopy and colonoscopy, now presumed to be of small intestinal origin. Though haemorrhoids remain the predominant cause for LGIB, this study has indicated the rising importance of diverticular disease, and marginally, colorectal cancer as cause of lower gastro-intestinal bleeding.

Some 80 percent of patients with LGIB experience spontaneous cessation of bleeding within 24 hours of admission, emphasizing the conservative approach to management; since patients with LGIB are generally in the older age group, the need remains to maintain a watchful eye for the twenty percent of patients that would need urgent resuscitation who may need surgical intervention.

Acknowledgement

I am grateful for the co-operation of the residents and my colleagues in the Departments of Medicine and Surgery as well as the contribution of the entire staff of the endoscopy centre in the collection and analysis of the clinical data presented in this paper.

References

1.   Eli, C. and May, A. Mid-gastrointestinal bleeding; capsule endoscopy and push-all-pul enteroscopy give rise to a new medical term. *Endoscopy*, 2006, 38:73-75.

2.   Rajo, G.S., Gerson, L., Das, A. and Lewis, B. American Gastro-enterological Association (AGA). Institute medical position statement on obscure of gastrointestinal bleeding. *Gastroenterology*, 2007:133:94-1696.

3.   Longstreth, G.F. Epidemiology and outcome of patients hospitalized with acute lower gastrointestinal haemorrhage; a population based study. *Amer. J. Gastroenterology*, 1997:92:419-424.

4.   Peura, D.A., Lanza, E.L., Costout, C.J. and Foutch, P.G. The American College of Gastroenterology bleeding Registry preliminary findings. *Amer. J. Gastroenteral* ,1997 92:924-928.

5.   Archampong E.Q., Badoe E.A. and Christian, F. Diverticular Disease in an Indigenous African Community. *Annals of Royal College of Surgeons England*, 1978 60(6) 464-470.

6.   Yoon, W., Jeong, Y.Y., Shin S.S. et al. Acute massive gastrointestinal bleeding; detection and localization with arterial phase multi-detectors row helical CT. *Radiology*, 2006 239:160-167.

7.   Holcomb, J.B., Helling, T.S. and Hirshberg. A military, civilian and rural application of damage control philosey. *Mil Med*. 2001: 166:490-493.

8.   Elta, G.H. Urgent colonoscopy for acute lower GI bleeding *Gastrointestinal Endoscopy* 2004:59:402-408

9.   Barnert, J. Messmann, H. Diagnosis and management of lower GI bleeding. *Nat Rev Gastroenterology Hepatal*, 209:6:637-646

10.   Barnert, J. Messmann, H. Management of lower gastrointestinal tract bleeding Best Pract. Res Clin. *Gastroenterology*, 2008:22:295-312

11. Lhewa, D.Y. and Strate, L.L. Pros and cons of colonoscopy in management of acute lower gastrointestinal bleeding 2012; *World Journal of Gastroenterol,* 18:1185-1190.

12. Levy, R. Barto. W. and Gani, J. Retrospective study of the utility of nuclear scientigraphic labeled red cell scanning for lower gastrointestinal bleeding. *AN2 Journal Surgery,*73: 205-209.

13. Howarth, D.M. The role of nuclear medicine in the detection of acute gastrointestinal bleeding. *Semin Nucl. Med,* 2006 36:133-146.

14. Farner, R., Lichliter, W., Kuhnj and Fisher, T.Total Colectomy versus limited colonic resection for acute lower gastrointestinal bleeding. *America Journal Surgical,* 1900; 178:587-591.

15. Stable, B.E. and Stamos, M.J. Surgical management of gastrointestinal bleeding. Gastroenterology Clinical North America 2000;29: 189-222

16. Baako, B.N. Diverticular disease of the colon in Accra, Ghana. *Br. J. Surg.* 2001;88:1595.

17. Lewis, M. Bleeding colonic diverticula. NDSG position paper. *Journal Clinical Gastroenterology,* 42; 456-1158.

18. Longsteth, G. F. Epidemiology and outcome of patients hospitalized with acute lower gastrointestinal haemorrhage; a population – based study. *America. Journal Gastroenterology,* 1997;92: 419-424.

19. Jensen DM, Machicado GA, Jutabha R, Kovacs TO, Urgent colonoscopy for the diagnosis and treatment of severe diverticular haemorrhage *New England Journal Medical,* 2000; 342:78-82.

20. Bokhari, M., Vernava A.M., Ure T. et al. Diverticular haemorrhage in the elderly - is it well tolerated? *Dis. Colon Rectum* 1966; 39 191-195.

21. Baum, S., Rosch J., Doller C.T. et al. Selective mesenteric arterial infusions in the management of massive diverticular haemorrhage *New England Journal Medical,* 1973; 288:1269-1272.

22. Milowski, P. J. and Schofield, P, F. Massive colonic haemorrhage – the case for right hemicolectomy. *Ann R Coll Surgical England,*1989:71:253-259.

23. Voeller, G.R., Bunch, G. and Britt, L.G. Use of technetium – labeled red blood, cell Scentigraphy in the detection and management of gastrointestinal haemorrhage. *Surgical,* 1991; 110:799-804.

24. Chaudhry, V., Hyser, M.J., Cracias, V.H. and Gau, F.C. Colonoscopy the initial test for acute lower gastrointestinal bleeding. *American Surgeons,* 64:723-728.

25. Lee, S. Wasserbrg , N. Detrone, P. et al. The prevalence of colo-rectal neoplasia in patients with end stage renal disease; a case control study. *International Journal of Colorectal Disease,* 23:47-51.

26. Nkrumah, K.N. Inflammatory Bowel Disease at Korle-Bu Teaching Hospital. *Ghana Medical Journal,* 2000. 34: 32-35.

27. Rajo, G.S., Gerson, L., Das, A. and Lewis, B. Review on obscure gastrointestinal bleeding. *Gastroenterology,* 2007, 133:1697-1717.

28. Thompson, J. N. Emingway, A.P., Macpherson, G. A., Reeshc, D. J. Spencer, J. Obscure gastrointestinal haemorrhage of small bowel origin. *British Medicine Journal,* 1984;288:1663-1665.

29. Veyradier, A., Ballan, A., Wolf, M., Giraud V., Montem Bault, S., Obert, B., Dagher, I., Chaput, J.C., Meyer, D., Navau, S. et al. Abnormal von Willebrand factor in bleeding angiodysplasias of the digestive tract. *Gastroenterology,* 2001; 120;346-353.

Chapter 12
Obstruction of the Biliary Tract
R. Darko

Introduction

The obstruction of the biliary tree may be intrahepatic or extrahepatic. It may also be partial or complete. When obstruction is significant the classical symptoms of jaundice, pruritus, pale stools and dark urine are prominent. Most cases of intra hepatic bile duct obstruction are not amenable for surgical repair and therefore emphasis will be placed on extrahepatic bile duct obstruction.

PREVALENCE OF THE DISEASE: The true incidence of the disease in Ghana is unknown but it is generally believed that carcinoma of the head of pancreas is the commonest cause, followed by a gall stone causing the biliary obstruction. The only paper published in West Africa was by Rahman et al. (2011) in which he described 64 cases seen over a 5-year period and found carcinoma of the head of pancreas constituting 60 percent of cases.[1]

There are many ways of classifying bile duct obstruction. The vast majority of bile duct obstructions are due to tumours or gall stones but the one classification that allows easy clinical identification is one that puts the cases into one of these four categories based on the behaviour of the jaundice.

1. Progressive jaundice: here it is common to find that the obstruction is complete and the jaundice becomes increasingly severe. They are all caused by tumour of the biliary tree except periampulary tumours. Included in this list is inadvertent ligation of the common bile duct and an impacted gallstone at the lower end of the bile duct.

2. Fluctuating jaundice: here the bile duct gets blocked and for a reason becomes unblocked again. The cycle then repeats itself. This is the typical behaviour of a stone in the common

bile duct which is not impacted. When the stone is impacted it gives rise to progressive jaundice. Other causes include periampullary tumours, intrabiliary parasites, choledochal cysts, duodenal diverticuli and papilloma of the bile duct.

3.   Chronic continuous obstruction: In this situation there is gradual stricture of the duct and usually does not proceed to rapid complete obstruction. This is seen in benign strictures of the bile duct. Other causes include chronic pancreatitis and stenosis of bilio-enteric anastomosis.

4.   Segmental obstruction: If only a few segmental ducts are obstructed since the liver has a large reserve, jaundice may not appear but the alkaline phosphatase will rise. The causes include tumours, injury and stones that involve only a few segments of the biliary tree in the liver.[2]

Pathophysiology of Bile Duct Obstruction

In the patient with bile duct obstruction there is hepatic dysfunction as well as systemic effects. With bile duct obstruction, the intrahepatic canaliculi become dilated and tortuous. The pressure in the bile duct is normally low (5-10cm of water) When bile duct pressure increases to more than 300mm of water, hepatic bile duct secretion ceases.[3] As a result the excretory products of the hepatocytes reflux directly into the vascular system resulting in systemic toxicity.

In the jaundiced patient, there is decreased capacity to excrete drugs that are normally secreted into bile.[4] High levels of bile acids induce *apaptosis*.[5] The synthesis of substances like albumin, clotting factors and immunoglobulins is considerably reduced. The Kupffer cell function, including phagocytosis, clearance of bacteria and endotoxins is considerably reduced.

Decreased cardiac function and reduced total peripheral resistance may make the jaundiced patient more susceptible to the development of post-operative shock than non-jaundiced patients.

Decreased cardiac function, hypovolaemia and endotoxaemia may be the leading factors in the development of renal failure in the jaundiced patient.

The increased levels of bile acids may be the cause of increased diuresis that occurs in biliary obstruction.[6]

Coagulation is impaired due to the reduced vitamin K absorption resulting from the lack of bile salts to aid the absorption of fat soluble vitamins.

Surgery in the jaundiced patient also results in reduced immunity leading to increased post-operative septic conditions.

There is an increased incidence of wound failure with increased incidence of incisional hernia in patients who undergo operation for obstructive jaundice. In bile duct obstruction usually there is dilatation of the portion proximal to area of obstruction. The degree of dilatation depends on the tissue that supports the intrahepatic bile ducts and how pliable the extra hepatic bile ducts are.

Physiology of Bile

Under normal circumstances 0.5-1.5 litres of bile is secreted each day into the intestine. Most of it is absorbed at the distal end of the ileum.

Bile has two main functions (a) it produces bile acids that are involved in the digestion of fats; (b) it excretes bilirubin, bile-soluble drugs and toxins. The inorganic component includes sodium, potassium, calcium and bicarbonate and their concentration is similar to their concentration in plasma. The major organic solutes are bile acids, bilirubin, cholesterol and phospholipids.[7]

When bile is not needed for digestion it is stored in the gall bladder as a result of pressure changes in the sphincter of Oddi, the cystic duct and the pressure in the gall bladder. In the gall bladder, water is absorbed with the resultant concentration of bile in the gall bladder. When the sphincter of Oddi relaxes, the little muscle in the common bile duct is able to push bile from the common bile duct into the duodenum. The action is aided by cholecystokinin and its analogues.

Biochemical Changes

Jaundice is the principal presentation of bile duct obstruction. Where the obstruction is incomplete, the jaundice may be marginal and where the jaundice is intermittent, repeated estimations of the bilirubin level are needed to detect the hyperbilirubinaemia. In obstructive jaundice it is the conjugated bilirubin which usually rises. In haemolytic jaundice it is the non-conjugated bilirubin that rises. In complex cases with prolonged partial obstruction of the biliary tract a mixed picture occurs and distinction between obstruction and other forms of disease may be difficult. In cholestasis resulting from mechanical causes the effect at the subcellular level is the same as the effect due to cholestasis caused by metabolic causes. This brings about difficulty in distinguishing biochemical differences between the two. In obstructive jaundice there is persistent absence of urobilinogen from the urine and bilirubin is usually present in the urine until there is significant hepatocellular damage.

Bile acid: The enterohepatic circulation will be interrupted when the bile duct obstruction is complete. This leads to increased urinary excretion of bile acids but not enough to compensate for the lack of excretion in the bile. There is also an increase in abnormal bile acid like ursodeoxycholic acid production. This type of bile acid is easily excreted in the urine.

The clinical presentation of obstructive jaundice includes pruritus and this is said to be due to the deposition of bile acids in the skin. Cholestyramine reduces the pruritus by sequestrating the bile salt in the bowel.

Alkaline Phosphatase

An obstruction of the bile duct leads to an increased production and hence the level in the blood. The elevation of alkaline phosphotase usually precedes the onset of jaundice. [8]

In patients with segmental bile duct obstruction even when the bilirubin is normal the alkaline phosphatase tends to be abnormal. In such a patient the alkaline phosphotase level tend to fall as the abnormal side atrophies.

A return to normal level after biliary tract surgery for obstruction is a good index of successful surgery.

The most common organisms are the usual bowel organisms and include E. Coli and Strept faecalis.[9]

In complete bile duct obstruction there is interruption of the enterohepatic circulation of bile salts and therefore the bile salts are not secreted in bile. The resultant poor digestion of fats will lead to steatorrhoea. The absence of the normal bile leads to a change in the flora of the bacteria of the upper part of the small intestine. The poor fat absorption leads to poor absorption of fat-soluble vitamins. Vitamin K_1 which is fat soluble, will therefore have to be given parenterally to minimize coagulation deficiencies. Bile salts bind endotoxin and therefore prevent its absorption from the intestine. Replacement of bile salts in the jaundiced patient may protect him/her against endotoxaemia.

Clinical Presentation of Obstructive Jaundice

The typical clinical presentation as shown by the patient with carcinoma of the head of pancreas is jaundice, pale stool, dark urine and pruritus.

There are various forms of presentation of obstructive jaundice. The four main types of presentation have been described and it is possible to clinch a diagnosis by putting the jaundice into one of these 4 categories. In obstructive jaundice due to malignancy, the jaundice tends to be progressive. When the jaundice presents with weight loss, the diagnosis tends to be easy. In late stages of the disease, there is usually an accompanying weight loss and perhaps the presence of a mass and lymph node enlargement. It must not be forgotten that an impacted stone in the bile duct and an iatrogenic bile duct injury may also present with progressive jaundice. In iatrogenic bile duct injury, the jaundice usually follows the operative procedure. Imaging has become the mainstay of diagnosis. The presence or absence of pain does not give away a diagnosis as pain does not distinguish between a benign and a malignant obstruction. The peri-ampullary tumour tends to present with fluctuating jaundice and intermittently palpable gall bladder. The carcinoma of the head of pancreas tends to present with constant enlarged non-tender gall bladder (Courvoisier's sign). Gall stones causing obstructive jaundice tend to present with pain due to the presence of biliary colic or acute pancreatitis or both.

A stone may remain in the common bile duct for a long time before giving rise to obstruction in the biliary tree. The jaundice tends to be fluctuating but occasionally it may be progressive when the stone is impacted in the bile duct. It may also present with cholangitis. The presence of fever and rigors and jaundice which represent the classical triad of Charcot is highly suggestive of choledocholithiasis. When this triad is accompanied by hypotension with mental confusion, it confirms the presence an acute, obstructive, suppurative cholangitis with impending bacteraemic shock.

Laboratory Investigations

The incidence of common bile duct stone is 8.6-18 percent.[10] Whereas unconjugated bilirubin may be elevated because of overproduction, decreased uptake and decreased production, conjugated bilirubin may be elevated as a result of decreased secretion, choleastasis and biliary tract obstruction. Bilirubin levels are neither sensitive nor specific for detecting liver disease. Because of the large functional reserve of the liver, the bilirubin level may be normal for a long time during progress of the disease of obstruction.

Alkaline Phosphatases

A high alkaline phosphatase level of liver origin usually indicates bile duct obstruction but will not distinguish between intrahepatic and extrahepatic bile duct obstruction.

The cytoplasmic enzymes, namely aspartate transaminase (AST) and alanine transaminase (ALT) may also be elevated in the early phase of obstruction and also due to infection and chronic obstruction. The elevation in chronic obstruction is an adverse prognostic feature. They are usually elevated in hepatocellular damage.

Biliary Imaging

Ultrasound of the Biliary Tract

Ultrasound is the initial investigation of choice in the patient with bile duct obstruction. The dilated ducts appear as tubules parallel to the portal vein branches and are known as the "correct double track sign" This is quite specific and characteristic of bile duct obstruction. Where a patient is examined immediately after the dilatation, this sign may be absent. In such a situation the ultrasound scan may be repeated after a few days. The level of obstruction can be defined by tracing the duct system down to the obstruction. When the obstruction is at the *porta hepatis*, there is dilatation of ducts in one or both lobes of the liver with a normal calibre common bile duct. When the obstruction is in the head of pancreas, the common bile duct together with the pancreatic duct are dilated. The head of pancreas in the "C" of the duodenum is difficult to scan because of the gas in the duodenum.

Various figures have been given by various authors as the normal size of the bile duct for example, Dewbury 2-5mm, [11] Cooperberg (1978) 1-4mm[12] and Behan & Kazam (1978) up to 8mm.[13]

When the stone is more than 5mm, it can usually be detected with an acoustic shadow. Smaller stones may not cast an acoustic shadow and are difficult to detect because they lodge further down the duct where duodenal gas may degrade the shadow. Small stones tend to lodge in the distal end of the bile duct and the gas in the duodenum may make visibility difficult. The semisolid bilirubinate stone may appear as soft tissue mass and simulate tumours. When a stone is impacted at the lower end of the common bile duct, usually there is some focal pancreatitis which may simulate a tumour on ultrasound.[14] Ultrasound may be used in the patient with obstructive jaundice in other situations such as intraoperative ultrasound to detect stone in the bile duct and in the post-operative setting to assess the bile duct.

Ultrasound may also be used to detect intrahepatic stones. Cholangiocarcinoma may be seen as a soft tissue mass extending along the biliary tree and it usually involves the adjacent portal vein but the full extent may be difficult to visualize on ultrasound.[15] Choledochal cyst is easy to recognize on ultrasound. Generally, ultrasonography is not sensitive to stones in the bile duct.

Computed Tomography of the Biliary Tract

There have been advances in the use of computed tomography (CT) in the field of the biliary tract. The data can be reconstructed into standard axial images or manipulated to display two-dimensional or three-dimensional reconstruction of the area of interest. After the relief of the bile duct obstruction, the calibre of the duct may remain dilated for the rest of the patient's life. In like manner, the bile duct may appear normal in an obstructed bile duct. CT may be used to identify the cause of obstruction. In malignant obstruction, the duct ends abruptly but in benign obstruction, the duct has a smooth tapering end.

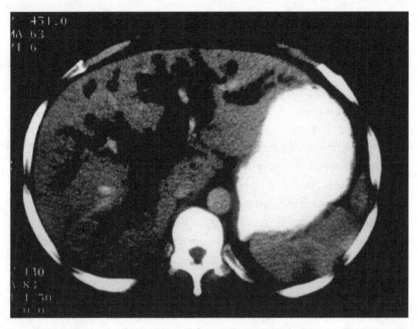

Figure 12.1: CT Scan showing Intrahepatic Bile Duct Dilatation

Magnetic Resonance Imaging of the Biliary Tract

Magnetic resonance imaging of the biliary tract is used to evaluate the biliary tract (MRI cholangiography) or both the biliary tract and pancreatic (magnetic resonance cholangiopancreatography – MRCP). MRCP therefore is the procedure of choice for diagnosis of common bile duct stones.

Treatment

When the obstruction is complete, it is easy to assess the outcome when the jaundice clears completely. When the obstruction is incomplete such an assessment is not so easy. This is particularly true of strictures.

Pre-Operative Preparation

In the jaundiced patient, if adequate preparation is not done complications are bound to occur.

Patients with obstructive jaundice often have anorexia and lose weight because of decreased oral intake. Other causes of malnutrition include malabsorption of fat and fat-soluble vitamins. The liver glycogen stores should be instituted by adequate intake of carbohydrates as well as daily infusion of 10 percent dextrose for 3 to 4 days before operation.

Coagulopathy that occurs in the jaundiced patient is corrected by administration of parenteral Vit K_1. The patient is given 10mg of intramuscular Vit K_1 daily for at least 5 days until the INR is about 1.3. To prevent post-operative renal failure it is important to ensure adequate pre-operative, intra-operative and post-operative hydration.

There is depressed immunity accompanying jaundice. Surgery in the jaundiced patient is therefore associated with a significant rate of surgical site infection. Antibiotic prophylaxis is required in the operation on the obstructed bile duct to reduce the chances of development of this surgical site infection.

The treatment involves removing the cause of the obstruction. The effect of treatment shows itself as clearance of the jaundice. Where removal of the cause is not possible, the point of obstruction is bypassed or stented.

Choledocholithiasis

In the past, the treatment of obstructive jaundice due to stones was open cholecystectomy and exploration of the common bile duct. With the widespread use of laparoscopic cholecysteomy, so many alternative have become available and many have challenged the open approach with exploration of the common bile duct as the first choice. The alternatives include precholecystectomy of postcholecystectomy with endoscopic retrograde cholangiography with papillotomy and stone extraction, laparoscopic exploration of common bile duct and percutaneous transhepatic extraction of the stone.

In patients who are unfit, or are elderly, endoscopic retrograde cholangiopancreatography and extraction of the stone is the preferred form of treatment followed by laparoscopic cholecystectomy if required.

The common bile duct is usually explored in about 15percent of all cholecysteomies and out of these, stones were extracted in about 65 percent of such situations. Open cholecystectomy with exploration of the common bile duct has a mortality of less than 2 percnt.[16]

In the fit patient, laparoscopic cholecystectomy is performed. The stone in the bile duct may be removed during the cholecystectomy of by pre-operative or post-operative stone extraction at ERCP. The advantage of pre-operative stone extraction is that if it fails, the stone could be removed during the cholecystectomy. On the other hand the complications of ERCP may also be avoided by performing cholecystectomy and exploration of the bile duct. Where an open cholecystectomy is necessary the exploration of the common bile duct may be performed at the same sitting.

Exploration of the Common Bile Duct

The site of the exploration of the bile duct depends on the site of the obstruction. However, where possible, the opening should be as distal as possible as most impacted stones in the bile duct occur distally. Another reason is that when it becomes necessary the hole in the bile duct may be connected to the duodenum. The duct may be palpated and the stone in the bile duct may be milked into the hole in the bile duct. Efforts should be made to ensure that all the stones in the bile duct have been removed. As the bile duct is irrigated with saline, small stone may float out of it. Another way of ensuring that the bile duct has been emptied is to insert a size 8 Foley's catheter or a Fogarty catheter and push it through the hole made in the common bile duct until it is in the duodenum. By controlling the filled balloon the catheter is pulled into the common bile duct. All stones proximal to the inflated balloon will be pulled proximally and directed out of the bile duct.

Where the duct cannot be said to be completely clear after exploration, choledocho-duodenostomy may be performed as the duodenum is close to the common bile duct. If that is anticipated, the choledochotomy should be done low enough to allow easy anastomosis with the duodenum.

After the exploration, a T-tube may be inserted through the hole in the bile duct to allow oedema and spasm of the sphincter to settle. Where this is not done, the distal end of the bile duct may appear functionally obstructed and lead to leakage of bile through the sutured hole in the bile duct. The size of the selected T-tube should be dependent on the size of the bile duct, usually, the bigger the T-tube the better. The lengths of the limbs to be left in the bile duct are shortened in order not to obstruct the duct. A T-tube cholangiography may be done on the table as a way of ensuring completeness of stone removal. The T-tube may also be used as the tract for subsequent removal of a retained stone in the bile duct. For this reason the limb of the T-tube that comes out should be as straight as possible. The free end of the T-tube is connected to a bag to drain freely and this is measured daily. There should be a continuous decrease in the volume in the bag as the bile continues to drain into the duodenum. A T-tube cholangiogram should be done at about the 7th day and if found satisfactory, the tube may be pulled out on day 9 post operative day.

Retained Stone

If a stone is found after the T-tube cholangiography, there are options of management. The patient may be sent home with a sealed drainage system. When the patient feels some discomfort the tube may be connected to a bag to drain the bile. After 5 weeks the cholangiography should be repeated. If the stone is still present, it may be removed by interventional radiology or by ERCP and papillotomy.

If by the 5th week the stone has dropped, then the T-tube should be pulled out gently.

If the stone cannot be removed by the methods described then it may be removed by a transduodenal approach with sphincteroplasty. With sphincteroplasty, the edges of the sphyinctorotomy are sutured to avoid stenosis and bleeding. The sphinctorotomy is made at about 11oclock position for 4-5mm. The initial longitudinal duodenotomy is closed transversely to avoid stenosis

Management of Obstructive Jaundice due to Carcinoma of the Head of Pancreas

Resection of the head of pancreas offers the best chance of cure of patients with carcinoma of the head of pancreas as it is the only treatment that gives the patient a significant a significant chance of longer surivival.[18] The median survival following resection is 14-20 months, while patients who do not undergo surgery due to advanced disease die at 4-6 months. 10-30 percent of those who undergo resection may survive 5 years.[18] The Kausch-Whipple procedure was named in honour of Walter Kausch and Allen Whipple, the two who pioneered the pancreatico-duodenectomy. The morbidity and mortality rates were quite high but since the 1980s they began to drop significantly. The reasons for the drop include improvement in diagnostic imaging, improvement in perioperative surgical support, and improvement in the surgical technique, particularly, the establishment of high volume centres. The mortality therefore is now in the range of 3-5 percent.[19] Other factors that have contributed to the success of resection have included vascular repair when invaded and extended lymphadenectomy.

Even though the TNM staging system is used in clinical trials, in practical terms most clinicians will like to know if the lesion is (a) resectable (b) locally unresectable or (C) metastatic disease.[20]

The Classical Whipple procedure involves resecting about 40 percent of the distal end of the stomach, cholecystectomy and removing the common bile duct, duodenum, proximal jejunum, and the regional lymph node all *en bloc*.

Pylorus-Preserving Pancreaticoduodenectomy (PPPD): The performance of gastrectomy brings with it certain complications. These include: gastric dumping, anastomotic ulcer and bile reflux gastritis. In the PPPD, the whole stomach, the proximal 2cm of the first part of the duodenum together with their neurovascular supply are preserved. There are many ways of handling the pancreatic remnant. Pancreaticocojejunal anastomosis may be performed in one of two ways. In one way the end of the transacted pancreas is inserted into the end of the jejunum. Another way is to anastomose the pancreatic duct to mucosa of the jejunum. Another way is to anastomose the pancreatic stump to the stomach. Another option is to occlude the pancreatic duct by suture or fill it with glue or some biologic material. This method has a high complication rate and is not encouraged. The gastrointestinal continuity is established by duodeno-jejunostomy by Roux–en-y by the antecolic route. The duodeno-jejunostomy should be 50cm downstream from the hepaticojejunostomy. Antecolic reconstruction is associated with fever complications more than retrocolic one.[21]

In non-resectable cases, biliary drainage can be achievd non-surgically by placing a biliary stent (endoscopic or percutaneous) or surgically by performing a bilio-enteric by-pass. The success rate for short-term relief of obstruction is comparable for surgical and non-surgical drainage procedures and they range from 80 percent to 100 percent.

Plastic stents may cause complications of migration and occlusion in about 40 percent of cases. Self-expandable metallic stents have a longer patency rate but they cannot be removed after placement.

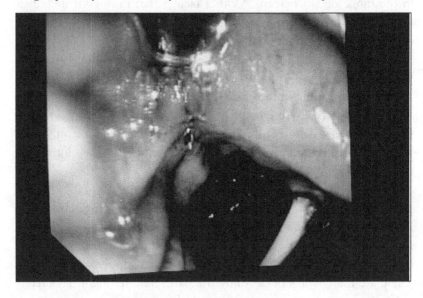

Figure 12.2: Carcinoma of the head of pancreas with the bile duct stented

A surgical bilioenteric bypass may be performed by anastomosing the gall bladder or bile duct to the jejunum termed cholecysto-jejunostomy and choledocho-jejunostomy respectively. Choledocho-jejunostomy is the preferred procedure because it has a better patency rate and lower incidence of cholangitits though technically it is more difficult to construct. The jejunal component may be a loop or a Roux –en-y. When a loop of jejunum is used ,a distal jejuno-jejunostomy may be constructed to prevent food from reaching the biliary tract (2-stage procedure) When there is an accompanying gastric outlet obstruction, a gastro-jejunostomy may be added (3-stage bypass) An endoscopic duodenal stenting is also an acceptable non-surgical procedure for the duodenal obstruction.[22]

Cholangiocarcinoma

Malignant lesions of the bile duct are not rare. The hilar area is the most common site. Cholangitis is a common feature of this disease. Diagnosis is by some form of cholangiograph. Where treatment is not possible, a bypass or stenting may be the palliative measure.

Post-Operative Bile Duct Strictures

Most bile duct strictures are due to iatrogenic injuries during operations of the biliary tract. Since the introduction of laparoscopic cholecystectomy there has been an increase in bile duct injuries. In open cholecystectomy, the injury rate is about 0.25 percent but in the laparoscopic era the rate is about 0.7 percent.[23]

Adjuvant Therapy

There is no satisfactory evidence for the use of chemotherapy or radiotherapy for surgically resectable tumours of the biliary tract.

References

1.   Rahman, G.A., Yusuf, I.F., Faniyi, A.O. and Etonyeaku, A.C. Management of patients with obstructive jaundice: experience in a developing country. *Nig Q J Hosp Med.* 2011 Jan-Mar;21(1):75-9.
2.   Benjamin, I.. S. The obstructed biliary tract. In: Blumgart, L.H. (ed.), *The Biliary Tract.* Churchill Livingston. 1982. 10:157-182.

3.   Lynn, J. A. 1979. Physiology of the extrahepatic biliary tree. In: Wright, R., Alberti, K.G.M.M., Karran, S. and Millward- Saddler, G.D.T. (eds.) Liver and Biliary disease: pathophysiology, diagnosis management. London: Saunders, ch 11, p 228.

4.   Blenkharn, J.I., McPherson, G.A. and Blumgart, L.H. Decreased biliary excretion of piperacillin after percutaneous orelief of extrahepatic obstructive jaundice. *Antimicrob agents Chemother* 1985 28;778-780.

5.   Patel, T., Bronk, S.F. and Gores, G.J. Increase in intracellular magnesium promotes glycodeoxycholate, induced apaptosis in rat hepatocytes. *J Clin Invest.* 1994;94(6):2183–2192.

6.   Green, J. and Better, O. S. Circulatory disturbance and renal dysfunction in liver disease and in obstructive jaundice. *Isr J Med Sci.* 1994 30;48-65.

7.   Blumgart, L. (ed.). *Surgery of liver, Biliary tract and Pancreas* 3rd Edition 2000 p 72.

8.   Blumgart, L. (ed.). *Surgery of liver, Biliary tract and Pancreas* 3rd Edition 2000 p 31.

9.   Darko, R. and Archampong E.Q. . The microflora of bile in Ghanaians. *West African Journal of Medicine* 1994 Vol 13 No 2 April-June 113-115

10.   Darko, R. The pattern of Gall Stone Disease in Ghana. 2nd Prof Victor Anumah Ngu lecture of the West African College of Surgeons Proceedings: WACS 2003.

11.   Dewbury, K.C. Visualization of normal biliary ducts by ultrasound. *British Journal of Radiology* 1980 53:774-780.

12.   Cooperberg, P. L. High resolution real time ultrasound in the evaluation of normal and obstructed biliary tract. Radiology 1978 129:477-480.

13.   Behan, M. and Kazam, E. Sonography of the common bile duct: value of the right anterior oblique view. *American Journal of Roentgenology,* 1978 130: 701-709.

14.   Blumgart, L. (ed.).Surgery of liver, Biliary tract and Pancreas 3rd Edition 2000 p636).

15.   Hann, L.E., Greatrex, K.C., Bach, A.M.et al. Cholangiocarcinoma at the hepatic hilus: sonographic findings. *AJR Am j Roentgenol,* 1997 168 985-989.

16.   Csendes, A., Burdiles, P. and Diaz, J.C. Present Role of classic choledochotomy in surgical treatment of patients with common bile duct stones. *World J Surg,* 1998 22:1167-1170.

17.   Wagner, M.R., Edwel, C., Buchler, M.W. .et al. Curative resection is the single most important factor determining outcome in patients with pancreatic adenocarcinoma. *Br J Surg,* 2004;91:586-594.

18.   Trede, M., Richter, A. and Wendel, K. Personal Observations, opinions and approaches to cancer of the pancreas and periampullary area. *Surg Clin North Am,* 2001;81:595-610.

19.   Beger, H.G., Rau B., Gansauge F. et al. Treatment of pancreatic cancer: challenge of the facts. *World J of Surg,* 2003;27:1075-1084.

20.   Haller, D.G. Future directions in the treatment of pancreatic cancer. *Semin Oncol* 2002 29 (suppl 20):31-39.

21.   Hartel, M., Wente M.N., Hinz U. et al. Effects of ante colic reconstruction on delayed gastric emptying after pylorus preserving Whipple procedure. *Arch Surg,* 2005;140:1094-1099.

22.   Holt, A., Patel, M. and Ahmed M. Palliation of patients with malignant gastroduodenal obstruction with self-expanding metallic stents: the treatment of choice. *Gastrointest Endosc,* 2004 60:1010-1017.

23.   Schol, F.P., Go, P.M. and Gouma D.J. Risk factors for bile duct injuries in laparoscopic cholecystectomy: analysis of 49 cases. *Br j Surg,* 1995;82:565-6.

Chapter 13
Lower Urinary Tract Obstruction
M. Y. Kyei

Introduction

Lower urinary tract obstruction (LUTO) refers to conditions that may block the flow of urine from the bladder leading to difficulty with voiding and associated poor urinary stream.

The lower urinary tract, comprising the bladder and urethra, acts as a functional unit that allows low pressure storage of urine and subsequent emptying (i.e. voiding) at intervals when appropriate. The urinary bladder acts as a reservoir for urine, storing the urine at low pressures. The first sensation of bladder distension occurs when the bladder gets filled with about 150mls of urine. However, voluntary control through the pontine micturition centre allows further storage to about 300-450mls of urine. Thereafter, there is an intense desire to void that causes the spinal micturition reflex to override that of the voluntary control leading to spontaneous voiding.

At the time of voiding, there is contraction of the detrusor (or bladder) muscles, relaxation of the bladder neck and the external urethral sphincter allowing urine to flow. Urethral distention which results from the flow of urine through the urethra stimulates stretch receptors in the urethral wall which reflexly reinforce detrusor contraction and facilitate complete bladder emptying (urethrovesical reflex).[1]

In the presence of poor bladder contraction, abnormal sphincter function (i.e. non-relaxation) and anatomic obstructions, urine flow is impeded, leading to the symptoms and signs of lower urinary tract obstruction.

LUTO results in the development of some secondary changes in the bladder. These include hypertrophy of the bladder/ detrusor muscles and increase collagen deposition in the bladder wall leading to the development of trabeculations and saccules. In severe cases there is the formation of bladder diveticula. The increase in intravesical pressure results in a back pressure effect leading to hydroureteronephrosis and subsequent renal failure.

Materials

This review considers primarily publications on various aspects of LUTO as have been undertaken in the Urology Unit of the Department of Surgery, Korle Bu Teaching Hospital. Reference has also been made to the preliminary findings of ongoing research work in the Unit. International publications as pertain to lower urinary tract obstruction have also been cited as deemed appropriate.

Causes

The causes of lower urinary tract obstruction include the following: benign prostatic hyperplasia, prostate cancer, urethral stricture and bladder neck tumours. It may also be caused by neurologic dysfunction emanating from disease or injury to the central or peripheral nervous systems such as spinal cord compression and radiculopathies due to osteoarthritis of the thoracolumbar spine and spondylolisthesis. The neurologic dysfunction may take the form of bladder weakness or incoordination between the bladder and external urethral sphincter, known as detrusor-sphincter-dyssynergia.

Generally, the causes of lower urinary tract obstruction show some variation according to age. The Ghanaian experience is also in support of this assertion.

Urethral strictures

Urethral stricture is the narrowing and loss of distensibility of the urethra resulting from fibrosis which may be due to infection, trauma or malignancy. Rarely, it may be congenital in origin. Infection is the commonest cause of urethral strictures in Ghana. Trauma as a cause results from road traffic accidents and instrumentation such as urethral catheterization. The infective conditions comprise gonococcal and non-gonococcal urethritis. This is reflected in the fact that the majority of patients are relatively young.

The patients present with lower urinary tract obstructive symptoms which include hesitancy, straining at micturition, poor or weak urinary stream (or dribbling stream when severe), intermittency and feeling of incomplete bladder emptying. They also present with irritative symptoms such as frequency of micturition, urgency, nocturia and urge incontinence. Others may present with symptoms suggestive of complications. These include haematuria, dysuria or an intense spasmodic pain felt at or just after micturition; they are usually secondary to urinary tract infection or bladder/urethral calculi. Acute urinary retention (i.e. inability to pass urine despite the urge and in the presence of painful distended bladder) is also a common mode of presentation. On physical examination the following signs, some of which are also complications of urethral stricture, may be found, namely: urethral induration, paraurethral abscess and urethrocutaneous fistula. Examination may also show a grossly swollen scrotum, the result of extravasation of urine, which may progress to Fournier's gangrene.

The passage of a urethral catheter is unsuccessful in the presence of a urethral stricture, with the catheter being arrested at the site of the stricture. In patients presenting with acute retention of urine, a stab suprapubic cystostomy is done to insert a catheter into the bladder in order to relieve the urinary retention. This also facilitates further assessment of the extent of the stricture.

Retrograde urethrogram remains a very useful investigation in the diagnosis of urethral strictures. It will show the stricture to be either partial or complete, single or multiple as well as the location of the stricture(s) in the urethra. (Figure13.1).

Any associated complications such as urethrocutaneous fistulae are also seen.

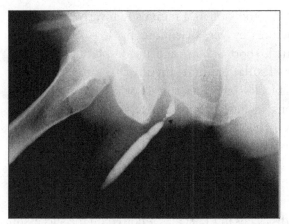

Figure 13.1: Bulbar urethral stricture shown in a urethrogram (Arrow head)

In the presence of a complete urethral stricture, the presence of suprapubic catheter from prior suprapubic cystostomy allows the performance of a micturiting/ voiding cystourethrogram that allows the determination of the length of the stricture. A urethral stricture may also be diagnosed endoscopically with a urethrocystoscope.

Abdominopelvic ultrasound allows the determination of post-void residual urine volume and also the presence of a complicating hydroureteronephrosis. Uroflowmetry, with the determination of the peak flow rate, the average urine flow rate and the duration of micturition, allows an objective assessment of the extent of obstruction. A peakflow rate of less than 10ml/s indicates significant lower urinary tract obstruction by the stricture.

The definitive management of urethral strictures is dependent on the characteristics of the stricture(s). The options for definitive treatment include urethral dilatation, visual/optical internal urethrotomy and urethroplasty. The latter could be either anastomotic or substitution urethroplasty. Strictures amenable to urethral dilatation should be partial / passable strictures and short in length. This approach is usually preferred in patients who are poor surgical risks due to the presence of significant co-morbidities. It has the disadvantage of early recurrence of the stricture and it can be complicated through creation of false passages, urethral bleeding and urinary tract infection.

Visual internal urethrotomy offers a minimally invasive method of treating urethral strictures by way of endoscopy. It is indicated for the treatment of partial, short (<2cm) and uncomplicated (e.g. free of a urethrocutaneous fistula) urethral strictures. The procedure can be done with a glans block, spinal anaesthesia or general anaesthesia. Possible complications include creation of false passages, urethral bleeding, urinary incontinence and rarely erectile dysfunction from injury to the cavernosal bodies.

In a series of 51 cases done under local anaesthesia reported by Klufio and Quartey,[2] the success rate after internal urethrotomy for urethral strictures was 84.6 percent after a follow-up period of between 3 months to 15 months. Mensah J.E. et al. [3] reported on the successful use of glans block for visual internal urethrotomy. In a recent series from the same centre, 190 patients with urethral strictures were also treated by visual internal urethrotomy. Their mean age was 52.5 years. The cause of the urethral stricture was found to be due to the following: infection - 90.5 percent, trauma -6.8 percent and iatrogenic such as urethral catheterization - 3.7 percent. The treatment was unsuccessful in 9.5 percent of the patients who therefore underwent urethroplasty subsequently (*Unpublished data*).

Urethroplasty is the treatment of choice for complete urethral strictures as well as long or multiple strictures. It is also indicated in the presence of complications like urethrocutaneous fistula and in relatively young patients as urethral stricture recurrence is high. Anastomotic urethroplasty is appropriate in the presence of anterior urethral strictures less than 2.5cm in length and located in the bulbar region, and also for posterior urethral strictures (i.e. those involving the membranous and prostatic urethra). Bulbar strictures longer than 2.5cm and strictures located in the penile urethra are best managed by substitution urethroplasty. The methods of substitution urethro-plasty include the use of penile skin flaps as described by Quartey,[4] and now called Quartey urethroplasty, the bladder mucosa and the buccal mucosa. Also described is the use of skin grafts. In our centre, Quartey's penile skin flap and buccal mucosal graft are the standard techniques of substitution urethroplasty generally used. Prof

J.K.Quartey is celebrated for his research on the microvasculature of the penile skin; the basis for successful substitution urethroplasty.

Benign Prostate Hyperplasia

The prostate gland is located below the bladder and is traversed by the prostatic urethra. The prostate causes obstruction to the urine flow by dynamic and adynamic forces. The dynamic obstruction is due to the contraction of the smooth muscles in the prostate resulting in increased resistance to urine flow, at the level of the prostatic urethra. The smooth muscles are under the influence of alpha-adrenergic nerves which when stimulated cause the smooth muscles to contract and thus impede urine flow. The adynamic (or static) component is due to the glandular and stromal component of the prostate which also reflect thes size or weight of the prostate. The development of benign prostatic (BPH) hyperplasia has been attributed to the effect of intraprostatic growth factors which are extrinsically influenced by the changing oestrogen and androgen levels that occur in ageing men and adrenergic signaling leading to a predominantly fibromuscular hyperplasia and the lower urinary symptoms observed.[5] Their presenting symptoms include obstructive symptoms such as straining at micturition, poor urine flow, intermittency, hesitancy and dribbling of urine. They may also have irritative symptoms such as nocturia, frequency and urgency. Some of the patients present with complications such as acute retention of urine which has been observed as the commonest cause of acute retention of urine at the Korle Bu Teaching Hospital.[6]The prostate, on digital rectal examination, is found to be firm, smooth, well defined, and with intact median sulcus.

In the evaluation of a patient with BPH, the international prostate symptom score (IPSS) evaluates the patient's experience with each of seven of the lower urinary symptoms over the previous month, on a scale of 0 to 5 (in ascending order of severity). The symptoms assessed include four obstructive symptoms, namely straining at micturition, weak urine stream, intermittency and feeling of incomplete bladder emptying together with three irritative symptoms, namely frequency of micturition, urgency and nocturia. Patients with scores 0-7 have minimal symptoms, 8-19 moderate symptoms and 20-35 severe symptoms. Also assessed is the single quality of life question which is assigned a score of 0-6. While patients who score 2 or below are generally happy with voiding, those who score 3-6 are bothered by their symptoms and need intervention.

In a study by Chokkalingam et al.,[7] on the age-standardized prevalence of BPH and/or LUTS among West Africans, they concluded that although there was no universally agreed-upon definition of BPH/LUTS thus making comparisons across populations difficult, BPH and/or LUTS appeared to be quite common among older Ghanaian men and that after age standardization, the prevalence of DRE-detected enlarged prostate in Ghanaian men was higher than previously reported for American men, but the prevalence of LUTS was lower than previously reported for African Americans.

Uroflowmetry, which assesses the strength of urine flow, is also determined. A maximum or peak urine flow rate of 10ml/s or less is found in 90 percent of patients with LUTO,[8] while those with scores above 15ml/s have good urine flow. Though a complete urodynamic assessment has been indicated as the gold standard for the assessment of bladder outlet obstruction in order to differentiate between outlet obstruction and detrusor underactivity,[9] uroflowmetry is the test currently available in our centre. A residual urine volume after voiding greater than 100mls indicates possible obstruction to urine flow though it has been observed that it weakly correlates with obstruction.[10]

In a series of 566 Ghanaian patients with symptoms due to benign prostatic hyperplasia reported by Kyei et al.,[11] the following results were obtained: the mean patient age was 62.8± 9.2 years; 32.5 percent had mild symptoms, 51.1 percent moderate symptoms, and 16.4 percent had severe symptoms. With regards to bothersome symptoms; 69.9 percent were bothered by their symptoms with the single quality of life scores ≥ 3; There was a strong positive correlation between the IPSS score and the single quality of life (QOL) score (p<.001), the post-void residual urine volume (p<.001) and the transrectal prostate volume (p<.001) but a strong negative correlation to the peak flow rate (p<-.001). It was concluded that the strength of the correlation supported the assertion that these parameters are best assessed independently in the decision making in patients presenting with lower urinary tract obstruction due to prostate enlargement.

The treatment of BPH is currently mostly medical. This includes the use of alpha adrenergic blockers like terazosin, tamsulosin and alfuzosin which have selective action on the smooth muscles of the bladder neck and prostate. They have the effect of relaxing these smooth muscles, leading to improved urine flow. Five-alpha reductase inhibitors (5-ARIs) such as finasteride have the effect of reducing the glandular component of the prostate and hence causing shrinkage of the prostate with associated improvement in urine flow. While the effect of the alpha blockers may be noticed within a few days, the response to 5-ARIs may take 3- 6 months to get to its maximum.

The surgical management of BPH is indicated when it produces complications. These include refractory (repeated) retention of urine which remains the commonest indication for the surgical management of BPH.(Figure 13.2)

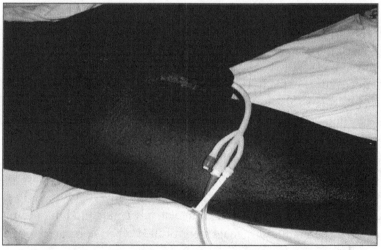

Figure 13.2: A patient with urethral catheter in situ for acute retention of urine

Other indications include the development of haematuria,(Figure 13.3) bladder calculi, diverticula, and impaired renal function as a result of persistent obstruction to urine flow.

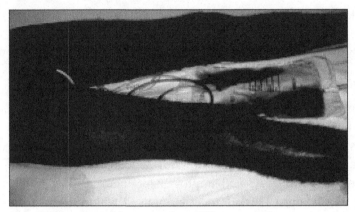

Figure 13.3 A patient with haematuria due to BPH

Patients who are unable to tolerate medical therapy as a result of side effects such as postural hypotension and headaches are also offered surgical management.

The surgical options include minimally invasive procedures such as transurethral needle ablation of the prostate (TUNA), laser therapies which include ablation therapies, resection and enucleation of the prostate and electrocautery transurethral resection of the prostate (TURP). These procedures are usually used for prostates that are relatively small. TURP is currently being used for prostates up to 75g due to the introduction of the bipolar resectoscope using normal saline as the irrigation fluid with less risk of the transurethral resection syndrome (TUR syndrome). Open surgical procedures used in the management of BPH include transvesical and retropubic prostatectomies. These are used in the setting of either large prostates or BPH with associated large bladder calculi or diverticulum. Various studies have confirmed that there is a relatively better and long-lasting effect after open surgical management of BPH when compared to the minimally invasive methods.[12]

In a series of 58 patients who had surgical management of BPH at the Urology Unit of the Department of Surgery, Korle Bu Teaching Hospital, 79.3 percent had open prostatectomy while 20.7 percent had TURP. The mean age of the patients was 70.4 ± 10.2 years with the commonest clinical indication being refractory retention of urine (76 percent). It was concluded that access to TURP in the surgical management of BPH in Ghana was low as it was observed that with improved facilities including routine use of transrectal ultrasound (TRUS) scan for assessing prostate size and availability of expertise for TURP, 67.4 percent of patients offered open prostatectomy presently could benefit from TURP, using prostate volumes 75mls (75g) or less as indication for TURP.[13]

Prostate cancer remains one of the common causes of LUTO in the male population. It is also the commonest internal organ malignancy in males. In Ghana it is the second commonest cause of cancer death in males.[14] The cause of prostate cancer remains unknown, however , risk factors noted to contribute towards its occurrence include aging and the African race. Genetic factors have also been noted to account for about 10-16 percent of prostate cancers.[15,16]

Prostatic infection is suspected to be a risk factor for prostate cancer.[17] Other probable risk factors include high intake of red meat, dietary fat (especially saturated) as well as calcium. Obesity, smoking and alcohol intake have also been noted to increase the risk of developing prostate cancer.

Screening for prostate cancer using the prostate specific antigen, has increased the numbers of prostate cancers detected incidentally, with its clinical significance still being investigated.[18] Symptomatic patients may present with obstructive and irritative lower urinary tract symptoms as well as haematuria (blood in the urine). In a locally advanced disease, symptoms related to erectile function observed include erectile dysfunction, haematospermia and painful ejaculation. In the presence of metastasis, the patients may present with low back pain, paraparesis or paraplegia due to the involvement of the lumbar and sacral spine. A combination of the patient's symptoms and findings on physical examination including DRE (hard, irregular surface and obliterated median sulcus) would suggest a clinical diagnosis of prostate cancer.

Prostate cancer is confirmed histologically by transrectal ultrasound -guided biopsy of the prostate. The commonest histological type of prostate cancer encountered is the adenocarcinoma which forms about 98 percent of the cases. Since the tumour is generally heterogeneous the grade is reported as a Gleason score. This system examines the first and second most predominant histological patterns and grades each on a scale of 1 to 5. The sum of the two grades produces the Gleason score. Patients with a score less than 7 have a well differentiated tumour; a score of 7 means intermediate and a score of 8-10 means poorly differentiated tumours. The latter have associated high risk of metastasis and treatment failure.

The definitive treatment of prostate cancer depends on the stage of the prostate cancer at the time of diagnosis. For a cancer confined to the prostate/ localized tumour, the treatment options include radical prostatectomy, brachytherapy and external beam radiotherapy. High-intensity focused ultrasound (HIFU) is also increasingly used in selected patients with localized prostate cancer.

Radical prostatectomy involves the surgical removal of the prostate and the seminal vesicles (Figure 13.4) with related pelvic lymph nodes and the anastomosis of the bladder neck to the membranous urethra.

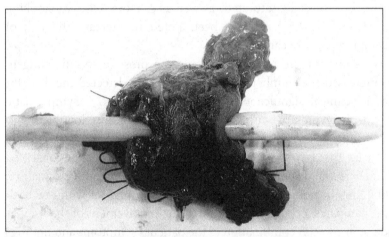

Figure 13.4: A radical prostatectomy specimen of the prostate and attached seminal vesicles

The procedure can be done either transperineally or retropubically. The major complications associated with radical prostatectomy include peri-operative haemorrhage, urinary incontinence, bladder neck stenosis and erectile dysfunction. A careful securing of the dorsal vein complex helps reduce the intra-operative haemorrhage and a mucosa-to-mucosa anastomosis of the bladder neck to the membranous urethra and the preservation of an adequate length of the membranous urethra help avoid urinary incontinence and anasto-motic strictures. In the absence of prostatic capsular extension of the cancer a bilateral or unilateral nerve sparing procedure helps maintain penile erections after radical retropubic prostatectomy.

Analysis of a series of 13 patients who underwent radical retropubic prostatectomy for localized prostate cancer at our centre recently produced the following preliminary results: mean patient age was 62.1 ± 4.9 years ; 46.1 percent presented with lower urinary tract symptoms, 23.1 percent with refractory retention of urine and the rest were asymptomatic (screening detected); pre-operatively 69.2 percent (9/13) had normal potency, out of which 77.8 percent (7/9) maintained their potency; one patient (7.7 percent) developed urinary incontinence (*Unpublished data*).

Intestitial brachytherapy involves the placement of radioactive seeds into the prostate under ultrasound guidance and this irradiates the prostate leading to the cure of the prostate cancer.

External beam radiotherapy is also used in the treatment of a localized prostate cancer. With the introduction of the linear accelerator and intensity modulated radiation therapy, fewer side effects are observed.

Patients with locally advanced prostate cancers are managed with a combination of either radical prostatectomy with antiandrogens or external beam radiation therapy with antiandrogens. These combina-tions offer a longer disease-free survival than surgery or radiation alone.

In the case of patients with metastatic prostate cancer, hormonal treatment is used. This include performing bilateral total orchidectomy, the use of antiandrogens such as bicalutamide or flutamide, the use of a non-steroidal estrogen such as diethylstilboesterol or a leuteinising hormone releasing hormone agonist such as goserelin (zoladex).

In the presence of lower urinary symptoms, and a localized prostate cancer, radical prostatectomy with the removal of the obstructing prostate allows restoration of good urinary flow. Radiation therapy can be used after an initial TURP as this therapy tends to worsen the lower urinary symptoms. The use of hormonal therapy in locally advanced and metastatic prostate cancer leads to apoptosis of the malignant cells and a resultant decrease in prostate size which results in improved urine flow rate. In patients with acute retention of urine, a temporary placement of urethral catheter and a subsequent trial of micturition without the catheter is carried out; if unsuccessful a TURP is done.

In the paediatric age group, the presence of posterior urethral valves in males remains one of the common causes of LUTO. While phimosis is common in some regions, in Ghana due to a high rate of infant/childhood circumcision it remains uncommon.

Posterior urethral valves are located in the posterior urethra and develop at the point of incorporation of the distal Wolffian ducts to the cloaca. These valve-like leaflets come together during voiding and obstruct the flow of urine. This results in thickening of the bladder wall from hypertrophy and hyperplasia of the detrusor muscles and increaseD collagen deposition in the bladder wall, leading to increased intravesical pressure with associated hydroureteronephrosis. Posterior urethral valves develop *in utero* and patients may be born with grossly distended bladder and renal insufficiency that in severe cases may be incompatible with life. Patients with minimally obstructing valves may present in childhood with recurrent urinary tract infections, failure to thrive, and lethargy and lower urinary tract obstructive symptoms. Examination will reveal patients with stunted growth, and distended bladder from chronic retention of urine. Palpable kidneys are found in the presence of gross hydroureteronephrosis. The diagnostic test of choice is micturiting cysto-urethrogram that will show gross distended bladder or bladder wall hypertrophy with trabeculations, saccules and sometimes diverticula. The classic findings include a dilated posterior urethra to the level of the posterior urethral valves that can sometimes be demonstrated and an associated narrow bladder neck due to the bladder wall hypertrophy. There may be vesico-ureteric reflux and reflux of contrast in to the ejaculatory ducts.

Other investigations include abdomen and pelvic ultrasound which will demonstrate the distended bladder and hydronephrosis if present. The renal function is assessed by determining the blood urea and creatinine level which, when high, is indicative of a poor prognosis. Radioisotope renal scintigraphy using either dimercaptosuccinic acid (DMSA) or mercaptoacetyltriglycine (MAG-3) will indicate the differential renal function and any cortical scarring or loss. The excretion rate can also be determined in MAG-3 studies.

Treatment involves urethrocystoscopy with fulguration of the posterior urethral valves. Vesicostomy is performed in babies or as a temporary measure in order to allow recovery of renal function and also allow a good size urethrocystocope to be passed for assessment and fulguration. Augmentation cystoplasty in the setting of increased intravesical pressure is done using either the stomach or ileum to increase the bladder capacity to protect the upper urinary tract and hence the renal function from further deterioration.

Phimosis is a condition in which the foreskin or prepuce cannot be freely retracted behind the glans penis. It is due to narrowing of the preputial opening. When the opening narrows to a pin hole it obstructs urine outflow. It affects the uncircumcised. They present with inability to retract the prepuce and/or lower urinary tract symptoms. The management is circumcision.

Paraphimosis is a condition in which the retracted foreskin cannot be reduced having become stuck behind the glans penis, constricting the penile shaft and causing vascular congestion and oedema of the glans and on occasions LUTO. It is managed initially with dorsal incision of the prepuce and circumcision when the oedema and any associated infection have been well controlled. In areas where the patients present early, reduction is attempted.

In the female population, LUTO is relatively uncommon. Although complaints of irritative lower urinary tract symptoms such as frequency, urgency and urge incontinence are not uncommon, they are often due to non-obstructive causes (e.g. urinary tract infection). In the presence of LUTO, classical symptoms of poor stream and straining at micturation will be obtained. The causes of lower urinary obstruction in females include inflammatory conditions leading to bladder neck fibrosis, meatal stenosis, and urethral strictures. Pelvic organ prolapse as observed in uterine prolapse, cystocele and rectocele are also common causes of lower urinary tract obstruction in females. Benign uterine fibroids and carcinoma of the cervix and vagina are other aetiological causes from extrinsic compression of the bladder neck and urethra or from infiltration. Iatrogenic causes from sling and other procedures for urinary incontinence are uncommon in our setting. Bladder calculi causing lower urinary tract obstruction have also been noted. Neurogenic dysfunction leading to lower urinary obstruction is seen in the setting of cerebrovascular accidents (CVA) and spinal injuries from road traffic accidents.

Though the diagnosis of LUTO has been made in women using videourodynamic studies with an obstruction being defined as radiographic evidence of obstruction between the bladder neck and distal urethra in the presence of a sustained detrusor contraction,[19,20] this is hardly used in Ghana. In our practice, diagnosis is based on symptoms, a careful physical examination including inspection of the introitus for atrophic vaginitis and urethral meatal stenosis, pelvic examination for pelvic organ prolaps such as cystocele, vaginal and cervical tumours and bimanual examination for pelvic masses. Post-void residual urine is assessed by ultrasound and values more than 100ml are considered significant. Cystoscopy may aid diagnosis when the procedure shows bladder trabeculations, saccules, or diverticula.

In the presence of atrophic vaginitis and associated urethral stenosis, urethral dilatation with the administration of oestrogen as replacement therapy or as oestrogen creams, pessaries and or hormone releasing- string have been helpful. The presence of urethral strictures requires urethroplasty which is challenging in females due to their short urethra, with urinary incontinence being a common complication of the procedure. Surgical repair of pelvic organ prolaps or hysterectomy is indicated in appropriate cases. Placement of a urethral/ suprapubic catheter or clean intermittent catheterization in the motivated is used initially for managing neurologic causes until recovery. Malignant lesions of the vagina and cervix are managed with either radical surgery or radiation with improvement of the lower urinary symptoms while myomectomy or hysterectomy is performed if the cause is uterine fibroids.

Conclusion

Lower urinary tract obstruction (LUTO) remains a major mode of presentation of patients in the Urology Unit of the Department of Surgery. While conditions leading to the development of urethral strictures are largely preventable, other conditions require not only well planned management strategies but also further research into more optimal and lasting interventions which are associated with fewer complications in the course of their management.

References

1. Shafik, A., Shafik, A.A., El-Sibai, O. and Ahmed Role of positive urethrovesical feedback in vesical evacuation. The concept of a second micturition reflex: the urethrovesical reflex. *World J Urol.* 2003 Aug; 21(3):167-70.

2. Klufio, G.O. and Quartey, J.K. Internal optical urethrotomy: a report of fifty-one cases treated under local anaesthesia. *West Afr J Med.* 1990 Jul-Sep;9(3):242-3.

3. Mensah, J.E., Quartey, J.K., Yeboah, E.D. and Klufio, G.O. Efficacy of intra corpus spongiosum anaesthesia in anterior urethral stricture. *African Journal of Urology* 2005; 2:111-114.

4. Quartey, J.K. One stage penile/preputial cutaneous island flap urethroplasty for urethral stricture: A preliminary report. *J Urol* 1983; 129:284-287.

5. Aeton, C.L. Aetiology and pathogenesis of benign prostatic hyperplasia. *Curr Opin Urol.* 2003; 13:7–10.

6. Yeboah, E.D. Acute retention of urine at Korle Bu Teaching Hospital. *Ghana Medical Journal* 1989; 19 (3):152-155.

7. Chokkalingam, A. P., Yeboah, E. D., Demarzo A. et al. Prevalence of BPH and lower urinary tract symptoms in West Africans. *Prostate Cancer Prostatic Dis.* 2012;15(2):170-6.

8. Abrams, P., Bruskewitz R., De La Rosette J. et al. The diagnosis of bladder outlet obstruction: urodynamics. In: Cockett ATK, Khoury S, Aso Y, et al., editors. *Proceedings, the 3rd International Consultation on BPH.* World Health Organization; 1995. pp. 299–367.

9. Nitti, V. Pressure Flow Urodynamic Studies: The Gold Standard for Diagnosing Bladder Outlet Obstruction *Rev Urol.* 2005; 7(Suppl 6): S14–S21.

10. Griffiths, D.J. Pressure-flow studies of micturition. *Urol Clin North Am.* 1996;23:279–297.

11. Kyei, M., Yeboah, E.D., Tettey, Y. and Kumoji, R. Correlation of prostate symptom score (IPSS) with quality of life, peak urine flow rate, post void residual urine volume and total TRUS prostate volume in Ghanaian men with LUTS due to prostatic enlargement. *Urology*. 2006; 68 (Supp): 105.

12. Misop Han, M.D., and Partin, A.W. Retropubic and Suprapubic Open Prostatectomy In: Wein, A.J. et al. (eds.). *Campbell-Walsh Urology*. Vol 3. 9th ed. Saunders Elsevier.2007: 2845-2852.

13. Kyei, M.Y., Mensah J.E., Gepi-Attee S. et al. Surgical management of BPH in Ghana: a need to improve access to transurethral resection of the prostate. (*East African medical journal* 63878-124141-1-SM.doc 2011.02-24.)

14. Wiredu, E.K. and Armah, H.B. Cancer mortality patterns in Ghana: a 10 year review of autopsies and hospital mortality.*BMC Public health* 2006. Jun 20;6:159.

15. Gronberg,H: Prostate cancer epidemiology. *Lancet* 2003; 361:859-864.

16. Ostrander, E.A., Markianos, K. and Stanford, J.L. Finding prostate cancer susceptibility genes. *Annual Review of Genomics and Human Genetics*. 2004; 5: 151-175.

17. Hrbacek, J., Urban, M., Hamsikova, E., Tacezy, R., Eis, V., Heracek, J. Serum antibodies against genitourinary infectious agents in prostate cancer and benign prostate hyperplasia patients: a case-control study. *BMC Cancer* 2011, 11:53.

18. Stangelberger, A., Waldert, M. and Djavan, B. Prostate Cancer in *Elderly Men Rev Urol*. 2008 Spring; 10(2): 111–119.

19. Nitti, V., Tu, L.M. and Gitlin, J. Diagnosing bladder outlet obstruction in women. *The Journal of Urology*.1999; 5:1535–1540.

20. Patel, R., and Nitti, V. W. Bladder Outlet Obstruction in Women: Prevalence, Recognition, and Management. *Current Urology Reports* 2001; 2:379–387.

Chapter 14
The History, Development and Future of the Cardiothoracic Unit:
Department of Surgery, College of Health Sciences, University of Ghana.

K. Frimpong-Boateng

Vision
The vision of the cardiothoracic and vascular surgery unit in the Department of Surgery is to be a world-class unit and first choice destination for management of cardiothoracic and vascular diseases in the West African sub-region and beyond.

Mission
Over the years the Cardiothoracic and vascular unit has remained a tertiary referral unit that has equipped its personnel with the requisite knowledge, skills and attitudes to undertake quality care, teaching and research at international standards to the ultimate satisfaction of its clients.

Values
The values of the unit are compassion, dedication, efficiency, sound ethical standards, punctuality, creativity and uncompromising integrity.

Historical Perspectives[1, 2, 3, 4]
For most of history, the human heart has been regarded as a forbidden organ too delicate to tamper with. Indeed the heart was considered outside the limit of surgery. In 1881, Theodore Billroth, one of the leading surgeons in the world, remarked: *"any surgeon who dared to operate on the heart would lose the respect of his fellow surgeons"*. In 1896, the usually perceptive British historian Stephen Paget wrote:

"*Surgery of the heart has probably reached the limits set by nature to all surgery; no new method and no new discovery can overcome the natural difficulties that attend a wound of the heart*". Ironically, on September 9 in that same year, Ludwig Rehn, a German successfully repaired a laceration of the heart and the first epoch in the development of worldwide cardiac surgery had begun.

A young gardener called Wilhelm Justus was stabbed in the chest in a park near the Main River in Frankfurt, Germany. He was found almost unconscious by the police and taken to the hospital, but not operated on until 48 hours later when his condition had deteriorated. At the operation he was found to have a laceration of the right ventricle. The bleeding was controlled with three silk stitches. Wilhelm Justus recovered, but developed an empyema (collection of pus in the chest cavity), which was drained on the 9th post-operative day. He eventually recovered and was discharged from hospital.

After 1896, there were reports of other suturing of heart wounds. For example, Rikketts in Cincinnati, USA, reported 20 successful cases among a patient population of 56. In 1908, Peck in New York operated on 140 patients with heart wounds and 45 of were successful. This was acceptable because almost all patients would have died without a heart operation.

Further milestones in the first epoch included the first pulmonary embolectomy which was performed by Friederich Trendelenburg at the University of Leipzig in 1907; the first widening of a stenosed mitral valve through a left ventricular approach by E.C. Cutter and S.A. Levine in Boston, USA in 1923. Henry Souttar performed the same operation through the left atrium in 1925 in London and the first successful operation of an aneurysm of the right ventricle by Ferdinand Sauerbruch in 1931.

The second epoch, which brought great strides in the development of heart surgery, was based on the understanding of the haemodynamics of the normal and the failing heart through pathologic, anatomic and clinical examinations with the help of cardiac catheterization.

In this respect Dr. Maude Abbott deserves special mention. Encouraged by her mentor and teacher William Osler in the Johns Hopkins University in Baltimore, she examined over 1,000 cases of cardiac failure in children and established the relationships between clinical symptoms and pathologic-anatomic findings. She thereby laid the foundation for the classification of congenital heart disease. Her book *"Atlas of Congenital Heart Disease"* published in 1936 aroused the interest of paediatricians in the English-speaking world.

Encouraged by the work of Maude Abbott, Robert Gross worked on the surgical management of patent ductus arteriosus (PDA) and in 1939 became the first person to publish closure of a PDA in 1939. The first closure of PDA, however, had been achieved in 1938 in Düsseldorf, Germany by Emil Frey on a 14 year old boy but he did not publish the case.

At about the same time, the paediatrician Hellen Taussig worked intensively to study cardiac failure in children at the Johns Hopkins University, Baltimore. Her work encouraged Dr. Alfred Blalock, who had moved from the University of Nashville, Tennessee, to Johns-Hopkins, to anastomose the subclavian artery to the pulmonary artery in children with Tetralogy of Fallot, a common and severe form of cyanotic heart disease (blue babies). This operation, performed successfully on three children referred by Taussig to Blalock in 1944, has been called *Blalock-Taussig Shunt* (B-T Shunt) and is still a useful operation in the palliation of many cases of cyanotic congenital heart disease.

The development of cardiac catheterization in 1929, in Berlin, Germany, by Werner Forssmann concluded the achievements in this second epoch.

The further development of flexible catheters which could withstand pressure, and the introduction of contrast media and the development of electronic equipment to measure pressure waves and blood gases made full-scale cardiac catheterization possible. André F. Counand and Dickinson W. Richards, who worked in Bellevue Hospital in New York, had since 1941 carried out extensive haemodynamic measurements using these new techniques. In 1956, these two, together with Werner Forssmann, were given the Nobel Prize in Medicine and Physiology.

The decisive breakthrough in the development of heart surgery to the stage we know it today occurred in the third epoch. This was largely due to the development of hypothermia and the heart lung machine.

In 1950 William G. Bigelow in Toronto, Canada, published the results of his studies on hypothermia. Bigelow showed that when the temperature of the body was lowered from the normal 37° C to 28° C, it resulted in reduction of basic metabolism and one could safely occlude the *vena cavae* to interrupt the circulation for about 6-8 minutes without significant injury to the central nervous system.

A few years later in 1952, F. J. Lewis, in Minneapolis, as well as H.C. Swan in Denver used hypothermia induced by surface cooling to perform open-heart correction of congenital heart disease.

In 1955, Ernst Derra, in Düsseldorf, Germany, employed surface cooling to close an atrial septal defect (ASD) for the first time in that country.

In Ghana, C.O. Easmon and his team used surface cooling to perform the first open-heart surgery in 1964, barely nine years after the first such operation in Germany, or, 11 years after the world's premiere in 1953 in the USA. Although Easmon performed only two such operation one of which was not successful, it must be remarked that, at that point in time Ghana was not too far behind the rest of the world, including such giants as the USA and Germany.

Because of the many disadvantages of surface cooling, researchers worked to find a way to replace the pump action of the heart and the gas exchange function of the lungs so that the heart could be stopped and worked upon.

John H. Gibbon from Boston has gone into history as the one who developed the pump oxygenator or heart-lung machine for clinical use. His experiments began in 1934. In 1953, Gibbon was able to close an atrial septal defect using the pump oxygenator to replace the function of the heart and lungs.

Several workers in different countries experimented with different machines. For example Senning and Crafoord in Stockholm constructed a pump oxygenator which they used in 1954 to do the first open-heart surgery in Scandinavia. They removed a tumour from the left atrium.

In 1960 Harken used the heart-lung machine to replace the aortic valve as we know it today. The following year Albert Starr performed the first mitral valve replacement using the ball-cage prosthesis which he developed with Edwards.

Ghana lost contact with the rest of the world of heart surgery in the mid-1960s. The heart-lung machine, which revolutionized open-heart surgery was not introduced in Ghana. It was about 30 years later that the author and his team, for the first time, used the heart-lung machine to perform open-heart surgery in Ghana. The first operation to replace a heart valve (mitral) in Ghana took place at the Korle Bu Teaching Hospital in 1992, 31 years after the world's first by Albert Starr in 1961.

One of the blessings in cardiology was the development of the principles of cardiac stimulation with electrodes as initially experimented by Hymann in 1932. Ake Senning and Elmquist, however, constructed the first implantable cardiac pacemaker, which was implanted in a patient in 1958.

The first pacemaker implantation in Ghana was performed by the author in 1989, another 31 years after the first ever such operation in the world.

Another important milestone in the development of heart surgery was the management of coronary artery disease. Initial attempts such as those performed by C. Beck (1935), Shaughnessy in London in 1936/37 and Lezius in Heidelberg, Germany, in 1938, consisted of attaching the greater omentum or lung to the heart so that collateral vessels could develop to enter the heart muscle.

In 1946, Vineberg in Montreal implanted the internal mammary artery directly into the myocardium.

The near-accidental discovery of selective coronary angiography by Mason Sones in 1962, in the Cleveland Clinic, Ohio, paved the way to the effective management of coronary artery disease. In 1967 Rene Favaloro, working with Effler also in the Cleveland Clinic, Ohio, performed the first aorto- coronary-artery-bypass with the saphenous vein as we know it today. In Ghana, the first coronary artery bypass operation was performed, again by the author and his team, in 1993.

A major problem in heart surgery was and is perhaps partial or complete replacement of the mechanical action of the heart temporarily or permanently. Heart transplantation, using the heart of a human donor, is at the moment the most durable replacement for the heart.

Basic experimental research was pioneered by Lower in Virginia and Norman Shumway in Stanford University, California. Christian Barnard went into history as being the first to perform successful heart transplantation in a human being at the Groote Schuur Hospital in Cape Town, South Africa, on the 3rd of December 1967. Soon afterwards Shumway performed the operation in the USA.

The first heart transplantations were followed by a proliferation of the procedure in many centres around the world but the limited success led to many centres abandoning their transplant programmes.

It was Shumway's group which carried out further experimental work and succeeded in establishing the basic requirements for a successful programme, such as diagnosis of tissue rejection through endomyocardial biopsy, immune-suppression as well as the selection of suitable donors and recipients.

The introduction of the immunosuppressant cyclosporin-A in the late 1970s as well as the introduction of non-invasive methods of diagnosis of rejection such as cytoimmunologic monitoring, brought a boom in the area of heart transplantation from 1980, so that in the 1980s about 10,000 transplantation procedures were performed worldwide.

Another area of cardiac surgery worthy of note is the replacement of the pumping action of the right or left ventricle or both. Kolfe and his colleagues Akutsu and Houston in Cleveland and later in Salt Lake City developed the first artificial heart in 1958. De Bakey and Cooley and Liotta also in USA, Bucherl in Germany and Nauratil in Austria also developed their models of artificial hearts.

Problems such as durability of the pumps and formation of blood clots on the membranes of the pump are responsible for the limited success of attempts at permanent total artificial heart programmes such as Jarvik-4, the artificial heart system, which De Vries implanted in Salt Lake City in 1982.

The development of anaesthesia, appropriate sutures, (especially the monofilament ones such as prolene), the electronic monitoring of patients and further improvement of cardiopulmonary perfusion have contributed to making open-heart procedures a reality today.

The practice of cardiovascular medicine in Ghana dates back to the early 1960s. In those years, Prof. Silas Dodu, an eminent physician and pioneer cardiologist, headed the Clinical Investigations Unit and started a cardiac clinic within the Department of Medicine of the Korle Bu Hospital.

With the assistance of expatriates such as Dr. S.K. Mitra in the Medical Unit of the Ministry of Health and Dr. M. Hawthorne, a medical physiologist on the staff of the erstwhile National Institute of Health and Medical Research, which preceded the Noguchi Institute, Dr. Dodu and his team ventured into the invasive field of cardiac catheterization. The Military coup in 1966, which brought about the exodus of most of the expatriate medical professionals contributed to the collapse of the cardiac catheterization programme.

On the surgical front, Dr. C. O. Easmon established a cardiothoracic surgical unit which together with trauma & orthopaedics, ENT (ear nose & throat), ophthalmology, was classified under 'Allied Surgery'. The surgical team, which also included Dr. Bannerjee, performed a number of chest surgeries including closed heart procedures such as opening of narrowed mitral valves.

Two open-heart procedures using surface cooling, that is putting anesthetized patients, usually children, in a bath and covering them with ice packs to achieve hypothermia, were also performed. Anaesthetic support was provided by Dr. Sen Gupta and Dr. K. A. Oduro. The initial pioneering work of Easmon suffered a setback after his retirement. The cardiothoracic unit became more of a unit for general thoracic surgery. This unit was run by Drs. Bannerjee and Mendes after Easmon's departure. Not long after that Bannerjee and Mendes also left the country.

They were followed by a succession of Ghanaian general surgeons who performed chest operations and limited closed heart procedures. The only exception was Dr. Seth Bekoe who trained as a cardiothoracic surgeon in the USA and who headed the cardiothoracic unit from 1975 to 1980.

The characteristic feature of the Cardiothoracic Unit (CTU) over the years was that a single surgeon at a time attempted to run the unit with no supporting staff. Diagnostic facilities to support the Unit were either absent or woefully inadequate. There were no dedicated wards and staff, especially nurses.

The initiative to establish the National Cardiothoracic Centre as we know it today dates back to about 30 years ago, in August 1981, when the author, then a staff at the Division for Thorax and Cardiovascular Surgery at the Hanover Medical School proposed the establishment of a modern cardiothoracic centre in Ghana.

This was an attempt to revive the pioneering work that was started in the 1960s by Prof. C.O. Easmon and continued over the years by a succession of surgeons including Dr. Seth Bekoe, Prof. Lade Wosornu, Prof. E.D Yeboah and Dr. M.P. Fitz Williams.

The breakthrough came through the efforts of the author and culminated in the establishment and commissioning of the National Cardiothoracic Centre (NCTC) April 1992. This heralded a phased development of cardiovascular medicine in Korle Bu.

In a university or teaching hospital the success of cardiothoracic and vascular surgery depends on a number of critical parameters such as training, staff, diagnostic facilities, equipment, space, organization and attitudes among others. No matter in which country (rich or poor) cardiac surgery is performed, standards cannot be compromised . There are standards of equipment, safety and comfort of patients and professional satisfaction of members of staff that had to be met.

Staff

The success of any cardiothoracic programme depends of the training of a host of professionals. A cardiothoracic surgical unit cannot exist in isolation. It needs inputs from others such as cardiologists, pulmonary physicians, anaesthetists, chemical laboratory scientists, microbiologists, radiologists, dieticians, physiotherapists, intensive care physicians, nurses, (including operation room, intensive care and specialized ward nurses). Other personnel include technologists and technicians who operate the heart-lung-machines and other heart assist devices as well as nurses and technicians who assist cardiologists in the cardiac catheterization laboratory. Secretariat services with all the modern modes of communication are also important.

The interplay of all these specialist functions in a coordinated, timely and efficient manner makes all the difference between success and failure and also between mediocrity and excellence. Nobody works in isolation and a true spirit of cooperation and interdependence must permeate the whole team.

In a number of hospitals, a lot of these departments (such as cardiology, anaesthesia, and laboratory) are independent but they are so efficient that their inputs into the cardiothoracic surgical service can always be relied on.

In most developing countries however, this efficiency cannot be taken for granted. This difference accounted for the challenges and difficulties that the pioneers of cardiothoracic surgery in Ghana, especially faced. With no trained supporting staff and efficient departments such as cardiology and aneasthesisa it was almost impossible for a lone surgeon, no matter his capabilities, to achieve the desired results.

It was to address the challenges faced by the pioneers of cardiothoracic surgery that the concept of a centre that would incorporate related specialties was proposed and implemented.

Training

The nucleus of the technical and nursing staff were trained in Germany in 1986/87 whilst I was still in Hannover. The team consisted of ICU nurses, intensive care nurses, perfussionists (technologists who operate the heart-lung machine and other heart assist devices).

When the centre started full scale operation in 1992 the training was extended to cover cardiac surgeons, anaesthetists and cardiologists(all within the fram work of the West Africa Postgraduate Medical College, as well as ICU and operating room nurses.

Phased development

Due to lack of funds, the development of the cardiothoracic unit took place in phases.

The first phase involved training of personnel (including cardiac technicians, ICU nurses, operating room nurses, laboratory technicians) and the bringing together of surgeons, physicians, cardiologist and anesthetists to form a cohesive team in pursuit of excellence. This phase also saw the acquisition of pieces of equipment and installations for both invasive and non-invasive diagnostic procedures. Infrastructure in terms of buildings and premises for equipment and other medical installations were inadequate initially.

The second phase, which was completed in 1994, saw marked improvement in infrastructure through the construction of an administration and diagnostic block and also the expansion of diagnostic facilities.

The third phase which was started in September 1998 involved the construction of wards, operating theatres, acute care unit, ICU and offices. Since the end of the third phase in 2002, all departments of the Centre have come to be housed under one roof, the present cardiothoracic block.

The Cardiothoracic Centre's first open-heart surgery utilizing the heart-lung machine and cardioplegic cardiac arrest was performed in 1992. The surgical programm has continued to evolve with the changing techniques and technologies that have made heart surgery in Ghana a safe and effective procedure.

Present Status of the Cardiothoracic Unit

The core functions of the Unit are teaching, training, research and service.

Teaching and Training

Five senior members -- four lecturers and a senior lecturer -- who were trained locally are staff of the Medical School.

Medical Students

Undergraduate medical students have been taught in the centre for several years. Batches of senior clerks come on rotation on regular basis. They also have access to the ward any time of the day throughout the year. Those in the pre-clinical years visit the centre regularly with their lecturers to acquaint themselves with physiological studies and measurements, including blood gases, in the intensive care unit.

Biomedical Students from the University of Ghana

Students from the Biomedical Engineering Department of the University of Ghana come periodically to the cardiothoracic centre for exposure to biomedical devices, processes and procedures.

Critical Care and Peri-operative Nursing

The practical training of nurses from all over Ghana who are doing the intensive-care and peri-operative care nursing courses sponsored by the Ministry of Health takes place at the National Cardiothoracic Centre. The centre is involved with the selection, teaching and final licensure examination for these nurses. The nurses also do their housemanship in the intensive care unit after their qualification. Several nurses from the West African sub-region do their attachment at the Centre. Over the past 10 years the centre has hosted about 350 nurses from West Africa, notably Nigeria.

Training (Sub-specialization)

The cardiothoracic unit has embarked on a programme of sub-special-ization. It is not optimal for one person to be operating on the hearts of adults and children and also performing other surgeries on the lungs, blood vessels, the oesophagus (gullet) and so on. For optimal patient care there has to be sub-specialization. One surgeon has specialized in thoracic surgery with special emphasis in minimally invasive thoracic surgery. Two others have specialized in paediatric heart surgery.

Another young surgeon is training in adult heart surgery. Another one has shown interest in heart transplant and heart assist devices.

Services

The cardiothoracic centre is the only place in this country where consistently since 1992, cardiac surgery, thoracic surgery, vascular surgery and intensive management, including haemodialysis, for seriously ill patients have been practiced at the highest level.

It is the only referral centre for patients with cardiothoracic and vascular disorders in Ghana and in entire West African sub-region. It is one of the few functioning heart centres on the African continent.

Research

World class research has taken place at the centre and its innovative work has been accepted worldwide thereby cementing the contribution of the Ghana Medical School to the world body of knowledge. Areas of research include the following:

- Management of patients with sickle cell disease undergoing cardiopulmonary bypass with hypothermia without employing exchange transfusion either before or during surgery.
- Management of patients undergoing cardiothoracic procedures, including open heart surgery who for one reason or the other (including religion) reject blood transfusion.
- Management of women through pregnancy and childbirth who have had heart valve replacement and are on anticoagulation medication.
- Trachea stabilization with autologous costal cartilage in acquired tracheomalacia.

Governance

Cardiothoracic care is complex and the governance should be handled with utmost care. The leader of the Cardiothoracic and Vascular Unit of the University Hospital should demonstrate the following characteristics:

1. Someone who can manage the human capital at the centre well;

2. That person should demonstrate sound academic credentials especially in research and contribution to the world body of knowledge;

3. Someone who is a good administrator;

4. A person of integrity with sound moral and ethical standards;

5. A role model for staff especially junior ones;

6. Someone who will encourage others to advance academically and professionally;

7. Someone who will have an ear for the social and other challenges facing members of staff.

The cardiothoracic unit in Korle Bu has a wide range of autonomy. This is necessary because of the inefficiencies in the Korle Bu system. However, in a well-structured and efficiently run university hospital, this autonomy may not be necessary.

The Impact of the Cardiothoracic Unit in Africa
On the Health Delivery System

1. The Cardiothoracic Unit with its present facilities and function is comparable to any such facility anywhere in the world. It has been accredited by the West African College of Surgeons as a centre of excellence to train cardiothoracic surgeons in the sub-region. So far this task has been executed creditably. Apart from Ghanaian surgeons, there have been surgeons from Togo, Nigeria and Ethiopia who have received training at the NCTC.

2. Regrettably there is only one true intensive care unit in Ghana and it is at the cardiothoracic centre. The ICU, apart from providing care for post-operative cardiothoracic patients and other critically ill patients, is also the training ground for nurses pursuing courses in critical care medicine and peri-operative patient care. Graduates of these courses can be found in all major hospitals in the country, providing high level patient care in their various locations.

3. The cardiothoracic centre in Ghana is one of the few functioning heart centres in Africa, providing cardiothoracic surgical services on sustained and consistent basis. Patients are

referred to the centre regularly from The Gambia, Sierra Leone, Liberia, Côte d'Ivoire, Togo, Benin and Nigeria. There are also occasional referrals from Ethiopia, Cameroon and Tanzania.

4. A large section of the international community in Ghana has found the cardiothoracic unit a place it can fall on, especially in cases of emergency. In the past, members of these communities were flown out without medical consultation in Ghana.

Cardiothoracic Unit and the National Economy

In the past, Ghana was able to sponsor less than a dozen people for heart and related surgery abroad. The cost of treatment abroad is high. On the average about $50,000 were spent on each patient. With the establishment of the Cardiothoracic Unit the number of patients who travel abroad for treatment of heart disease has drastically reduced. Savings from diagnostic procedures and management of non-cardiac conditions which hitherto were not performed in Ghana also run into several million dollars.

One cannot put monetary value on the satisfaction a poor and anxious child has when he receives medical care in his own familiar environment.

Foreign Direct Investment

Foreign entrepreneurs who decide to invest in developing countries have other factors to worry about apart from the basic economic parameters. One of these is their health and that of their employees. To most investors this is a very important consideration.

Because of the lack of adequate health facilities some investors, especially the large- and medium-scale ones, decide to set up their own health facilities. Small-scale businesses that may not be in a position to establish their own health care system. may look elsewhere to invest. The Cardiothoracic Unit over the years has had interactions with several investors and potential investors. These contacts might have in a way influenced the investors to do business in Ghana. Feedback from some of them, especially those in the mining, energy and tourism sectors, attest to the validity of this assumption. Patients from these establishments are regularly brought to the intensive care unit at the cardiothoracic unit either for management in Ghana or for stabilization prior to medical evacuation abroad. In this way the unit is contributing positively to the economic development of Ghana.

As a Model for other Centres

The performance of the Cardiothoracic Centre encouraged the government of Ghana to set up other centres of excellence in Korle Bu. Thus a high standard in health institution organization as well as training and management of hospital personnel has been set by the Cardiothoracic Unit.

Looking Ahead

Training and sub-specialization

From a sole surgical crusader and a few supporting staff 22 years ago, the staff strength has grown to over 130 people in all categories. It is particularly heartwarming that there are now six other highly qualified and motivated heart surgeons who are ready to keep the torch burning.

As more staff members are trained in cardiovascular care, sub-specialty training becomes a more realistic approach to attain cutting-edge efficiency. In 2008, Video Assisted Thoracoscopy Surgery (VATS) service was introduced. This system is a type of "keyhole" surgery technique that allows the performance of selected cardiothoracic cases without cutting the chest open.

Plans are already in place to establish a paediatric heart wing that will focus on care of children with congenital and acquired cardiovascular disease.

There is the need to train Ghanaian cardiologists who will be able to handle both non-invasive and invasive procedures, including electrophysiological management of arrhythmias and related disorders.

State of the art surgery

Worldwide there is a visible trend towards minimally invasive cardiac surgery, including robotic assisted surgery such as the da Vinci system for coronary artery bypass as well as laser transmyocardial revascularization and ventricular assist devices for end-stage heart disease. Since we cannot forever run behind the international community and also since our clients are becoming increasingly informed about surgical management modalities elsewhere, we should constantly keep our minds on training, skills update and acquisition of appropriate equipment.

Sub-regional cooperation

There is the need to look at sub-regional cooperation. No one country can do it alone, especially with regard to training and organ transplantation. There is the need to set up a sub-regional centre which will handle the database of all patients needing transplant so that when an organ is available in any country in the sub-region, any organ recipient in any country who matches the donor may receive it. Surgical teams may then fly to the country of the donor to harvest the organ(s) for transplantation.

Thus, what is suggested here is an ECOWAS TRANSPLANT facility with headquarters in Accra, much like the EURO TRANSPLANT for Europe with headquarters in Leiden, Holland.

Research

Unpublished research data indicate an increase in the incidence of dilatative cardiomyopathy in the sub-region. More research is needed to find possible causes, preventive measures and management including transplantation.

The mention of transplantation in West Africa should prompt research in the area of "growing human hearts" and other tissues for transplant using a process that will also involve stem cell research.

In this process the donor heart is removed from the body; pig hearts may also be suitable.

Detergents are then used to strip the cells from the heart leaving behind the protein skeleton or 'ghost heart'. Stem cells grown from cells taken from a patient are then added to the ghost heart in a bio-reactor. The stem cells then multiply and generate new heart cells which hopefully will beat spontaneously or with the help of pacemakers.

Cloning animal hearts (especially pig's heart) and other organs that will not be rejected by a human recipient will be another research possibility. All these procedures will be important in our part of the world where people want to go to the grave with all organs "intact"; in other words where people are not willing to donate organs.

References

1. A.P. Naef. The mid-century revolution in thoracic and cardiovascular surgery: Part 1 Interact CardioVasc Thorac Surg (2003) 2 (3): 219-226.
2. R. Hurt. The History of Cardiothoracic Surgery: From Early Times: August 15, 1996 | ISBN-10: 1850706816 | ISBN-13: 978-1850706816 | Edition: 1
3. K. Frimpong-Boateng. Deep Down My Heart, A history of Cardiothoracic Surgery in Ghana (2000):Accra:Woeli Publishing Services: ISBN 10-9988003986 ; ISBN-13: 978-9988003982.
4. William S. Stoney. Pioneers of Cardiac surgery: July 2008; ISBN-10: 0826515940; ISBN-13: 978-0826515940

Chapter 15
Management of Oesophageal Atresia in a Developing Country like Ghana
W. Appeadu-Mensah

Definition

Oesophageal atresia is a congenital abnormality in which there is a discontinuity in the wall or lumen of the oesophagus with or without an associated trachea-oesophageal fistula. There are, however, two types in which there is no discontinuity in the oesophagus but rather a fistula or a stenosis.

It has very good prognosis with early diagnosis and appropriate intervention.

Incidence

The incidence ranges between 1 in 3,500 and 1 in 4,500 live births world wide.[1,2]

In a retrospective analysis of cases seen at the Korle Bu Teaching Hospital in Ghana, 44 patients were seen over an 8 year period; 22 (or 50 percent) were male, 15 (or 39 percent) female while in 5 (or11 percent) the sex was not recorded. (Unpublished data).

Aetiology

The aetiology of oesophageal atresia is not known but a number of possible risk factors have been studied.[1,4,5,6,7]

Possible teratogenic risk factors include, Methimazole, Contraceptive pills, Thalidomide, and Diabetes. [4,5,6]

Genetic and chromosomal factors may play a role in a few cases but the majority are sporadic events with no clear-cut causative factor.[7] While some association with some of these factors has been noted no single factor can convincingly be said to cause oesophageal atresia.

Pathogenesis

The Pathogenesis of oesophageal atresia is not known but is suspected to be due to a failure of cellular proliferation, differentiation and apoptosis.[8] Damage usually occurs around the fourth week of gestation. During initial development, the foregut divides into the trachea anteriorly and the oesophagus posteriorly. It is at this stage that an insult leads to oesophageal atresia.

A number of proposed theories were summarized by Kluth and Spiegel[11] and these include:

Theory of foregut occlusion:

This theory suggests that there is a period of complete occlusion of the foregut followed later by recanalization. A form of failure of canalization is suggested to explain the pathogenesis of oesophageal atresia. In normal embryogenesis, a phase of complete occlusion of the foregut has never been observed.

Theory of spontaneous deviation of the trachea-oesophageal septum:

This theory proposes that during normal development, a tracheo-oesophageal septum forms which divides the foregut into an oesophagus and a trachea. An aberration in the formation of this septum is proposed to cause oesophageal atresia. An obvious septum has never, however, been observed during normal embryogenesis

Theory of mechanical pressure:

This theory suggests that during the course of embryogenesis ,abnormally high pressures develop which result in impaired formation of the oesophagus and trachea. It is, however, difficult to imagine high pressures at this early stage of embryogenesis.

Molecular Pathway

It has been shown that an aberration in the genetic pathway involving the sonic hedgehog gene may be involved in the pathogenesis of oesophageal atresia.[9,10]

Classification

A number of classifications have been proposed but the most useful have been those of Vogt (1929) [14] and Gross (1953) .[15]

The Gross classification is as follows:

Type A   Oesophageal Atresia without a fistula;

Type B   Oesophageal Atresia with a proximal Tracheo-oesophageal fistula;

Type C   Oesophageal Atresia with a distal Tracheo-oesophageal fistula. This is the commonest type encountered.

Type D   Oesphageal Atresia with double fistula;

Type E   Isolated Tracheo-oesophageal fistula;

Type F   Oesophageal stenosis.

This classification helps in accurate diagnosis of the type and helps plan the definitive management needed.

Associated Anomalies

Oesophageal Atresia is associated with other anomalies in about 50 percent to 70 percent of cases.[3] Not all, are life-threatening however. Association with cardiac malformations in particular is known to significantly affect prognosis.[12]

Known associations include VACTERL (Vertebral, Anorectal, Cardiac, Tracheo-esophageal atresia, Renal, Limb) anomalies, CHARGE (Coloboma of the eye, Heart defects, Atresia of the nasal choanae, Retardation of Growth/development, Genital and/or urinary) anomalies, Downs Syndrome and others. This may be due to an early teratogenic event that affects a number of possible organ systems.[8]

Pathophysiology

This depends on the specific type of Oesophageal atresia and any associated congenital anomalies. In the commonest type with a distal fistula, the child is at risk of constant aspiration of saliva and food from the proximal pouch. In addition, there is a constant risk of aspiration of gastric contents. Depending on how much air passes through the distal fistula, there is a risk of gastric dilatation which compromises respiration, as well as a risk of gastric perforation

Diagnosis

Diagnosis may be antenatal or postnatal. The timing of diagnosis significantly influences the management and prognosis. In most developed countries, diagnosis is currently made antenatally.[12] Ultrasound findings of polyhydramnios, an oesophageal pouch, a small stomach and delayed swallowing help make this antenatal diagnosis. The result of this is planned delivery at a centre where the neonate can receive appropriate care, investigations soon after birth and surgery, before there is a high risk of aspiration pneumonia. Many expectant women have an antenatal ultrasound examination done in Ghana but in only a few of them are congenital anomalies detected before birth. This could be due to the low resolution of available ultrasound machines or the large number of patients that are scanned by a single unit, thus not allowing enough time to properly scan each patient. In Ghana diagnosis is delayed due to late presentation. Children may present between the 3rd and 14th day of life with severe pneumonia, having already aspirated feeds, and with malnutrition which significantly affects the prognosis. In a review of patients seen at the Korle Bu Teaching Hospital over an eight- year period more than 50 percent presented after the age of 5 days. The surgeon must treat all these co-morbid conditions before embarking on surgery for oesophageal atresia.

In the post-natal diagnosis of trachea-oesophageal atresia, excessive salivation is the most important symptom and any child who is seen to require persistent suction soon after birth must not be fed. A radiopaque, nasogastric tube (size 8 to 10 FR) should be passed. Failure to pass the tube more than 10 cm from the mouth should be considered to suggest oesophageal atresia and an X-ray done to confirm this.

Failure to make the diagnosis at this stage results in feeding the child. This leads to coughing, cyanosis and choking after feeds which then become the presenting symptoms.The child develops aspiration pneumonia and may present with respiratory distress.

Examination reveals an ill child who may be preterm, in respiratory distress, with signs of pneumonia. The abdomen may be distended in patients with a distal fistula or scaphoid in those without a fistula.

Examination for other anomalies such as cardiac anomalies, anorectal malformation and hemi-vertebrae is undertaken

Investigations

A plain X-ray of the chest and abdomen confirms the diagnosis by showing the end of the tube in the chest (figure 15.1) and helps confirm the presence of a distal fistula by showing the presence of gas in the abdomen. A gasless abdomen on the X-ray will signify an atresia without a fistula (Figure 15.2). The chest X-ray also confirms pneumonia if present, gives an idea of the size and shape of the heart, and the presence or absence of vertebral anomalies. The abdominal x-ray may also confirm intestinal obstruction and show vertebral anomalies.

Abdominal Ultrasound is important for demonstrating any renal anomalies if present. Anomalies of the kidneys in these patients are not uncommon. In trisomy 18 in which children have no kidneys.

Echocardiography is an important investigation to identify cardiac anomalies. This investigation is routinely done in certain advanced centres because of the possible association with cardiac anomalies and it is of prognostic significance.[12] It is not routinely done in many developing countries including Ghana. Due to the large number of patients served by a single unit, echocardiography tends to be performed as an elective planned procedure. It is done when there is clinical evidence to suggest a cardiac malformation.

Contrast study of the proximal pouch should be avoided as much as possible since it often leads to aspiration of contrast. It must only be done in a tertiary centre by an experienced radiologist and in cases in which there is doubt about the diagnosis after thorough evaluation of the symptoms and signs. In the large majority of cases this investigation is not necessary.

Karyotyping may be necessary as a supportive investigation due to possible associations with conditions such as Down's syndrome and trisomy 18.

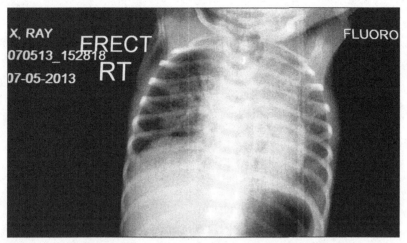

Figure 15.1: The tip of a nasogastric tube with Radio-opaque material arrested in the upper Chest. (arrow head)

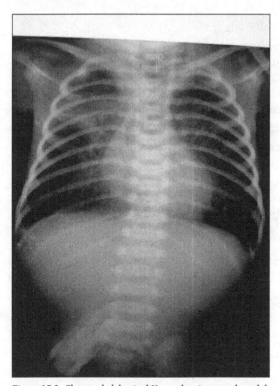

Figure 15.2: Chest and abdominal X-ray showing a gasless abdomen

Prognostic Classification

In 1962, Waterston [19] presented a prognostic classification of oesophageal atresia which became the main tool for prognostication. It was based on the birth weight of the baby, the presence of congenital anomalies and the presence of pneumonia. This classification helped predict significantly the prognosis in oesphageal atresia.

Waterston classification is as follows:

Group	Description	Survival Rate (%)
A	BW>2.5kg and healthy.	100
B	BW between 1.8kg-2.5kg and well OR Higher weight with moderate pneumonia/moderate congenital anomalies.	85
C	BW<1.8kg OR Higher weight with severe pneumonia/severe congenital anomalies.	65

With improvement in early diagnosis, intensive care for neonates, improved anaesthetic care and monitoring of neonates, survival in the advanced centres has improved and made the Waterston classification less relevant in these centres.[20] The Spitz [20]classification has, therefore, been proposed and found more relevant.

The Spitz classification is as follows:

Group	Description	Survival Rate (%)
I	BW>1.5kg with no major congenital heart disease	97
II	BW<1.5kg OR presence of major congenital heart disease	59
III	BW<1.5kg with major congenital heart disease	22

In this classification the only significant factors affecting prognosis are birth weight less than 1.5 kilograms and a major cardiac anomaly. With the ability to manage less severe associated anomalies adequately, these have become less relevant.

In the developing world the Waterston classification is still relevant because of late diagnosis which significantly increases the risk of pneumonia and malnutrition that bear on prognosis.

Treatment

In advanced countries where prenatal diagnosis is the norm, the most important prognostic indicator is the presence or absence of a major cardiac anomaly. In the presence of a cardiac anomaly, surgery for the cardiac condition may precede surgery for the oesophageal condition.[12,20] Prognosis is excellent for those without a major cardiac anomaly.[20]

Thoracotomy and primary oesophago-oesophagostomy is the management of choice. Long-gap atresias may be treated by delayed primary anastomosis or staged surgery.

Unpublished data from the author as well as data from the subregion indicate that presentation is late.[30]

The management of the commonest type (C) in this setting involves:

1. Admission and institution of immediate suction of the upper pouch at least once every 10 minutes;
2. Position of the patient in a gentle head up inclination to reduce the risk of aspiration of Gastric contents;
3. Antibiotics to treat pneumonia;
4. Intravenous fluids;
5. Injection of Vitamin K;
6. Maintenance of a warm Neonate;
7. Avoidance of unnecessary handling.

Surgery may be undertaken when pneumonia has been treated and any severe anomaly has been excluded; this may be difficult to achieve completely in the absence of adequate diagnostic facilities.

Options of surgery include: primary anastomosis, delayed primary anastomosis or staged repair.

Primary anastomosis involves thoracotomy, division of the fistula and an end-to-end oesophageal anastomosis.

Delayed primary anastomosis may be done after a period of time to allow resolution of pneumonia or after an initial thoracotomy to divide the fistula followed by a period of waiting until the child's condition has improved.[19] Patients who have no fistula may have a gastrostomy done with primary anastomosis later.

Staged repair involves a gastrostomy, oesophagostomy, division of a fistula and an oesophageal replacement when the child is older and can withstand a major abdominal surgery.[19,12] This is indicated in late presentations and in a small malnourished ill child when thoracotomy will be unsafe. The absence of ventilatory support for a small preterm baby may be an indication to do a staged procedure. In the developing world this is usually more common due to late presentation.[30] It may also be indicated in children with long-gap oesophageal atresia.

Complications

These include anastomotic leakage, complete dehiscence, stricture, sepsis, pneumothorax, gastro-oesophageal reflux, disordered oesophageal motility, tracheomalacia. The incidence of complications after late presentation and primary anastomosis is high.

Outcomes

Survival following adequate treatment has improved from 40 percent in the 1950s to over 90 percent currently in advanced centres.[12] In developing countries survival remains around 50 percent. In a retrospective study of patients seen at the Korle-bu Teaching hospital (unpublished data) 13 (40.6 percent) were alive, 18 (56.3 percent) died and for 1(3.1 percent) the result was unknown.

Conclusion

Oesophageal atresia is a congenital anomaly with excellent prognosis if diagnosed early and appropriately managed. Attempts to improve on early diagnosis would significantly affect the prognosis in developing countries. With the present state of facilities, the Waterston classification remains relevant in this part of the world and staged surgery may be more often indicated.

References

1. Shaw-Smith, C. Oesophageal atresia, TOF and the VACTERL association: review of genetics and epidemiology. *J Med Genet* 2006;43:545-554
2. Oldham, Colombani, and Foglia Principles and Practice of Paediatric Surgery, 4th Edition (2005):page 1040
3. Correl M. Congenital Anomalies of the Oesophagus. In: Grosfeld, J.L. et al. Paediatric Surgery, 6th ed. pg. 1053. Philadelphia, PA, USA: Mosby Elsevier.
4. zendrey, T., Danyi, G. and Czeizel, A.S. Aetiological study on isolated OA. *Hum Genet* 1985;70:51
5. Chen, H., Goei, G.S. and Hertzler, J.H. Family studies in congenital oesophageal atresia with or without TOF. *Birth Defects Orig Artic Ser* 1979;15(5c):117
6. Martinez-Frias, M.L. Epidemiological analysis of outcomes of pregnancy in diabetic mothers: identification of the most characteristic and most frequent congenital anomalies. *Am J Med Genet* 1994;51:108-113
7. Harris, J., Kallen, B. and Robert, E Descriptive epidemiology of alimentary tract atresia. *Teratology* 1995;52:15
8. Williams, A.K., Qi, B.Q. and Beasley SW. Temporo-spatial aberrations of apoptosis in the rat embryo developing oesophageal atresia. J *Pediatr Surg* 2000;35(11):1617-1620.
9. Vleesch Dubois, V. N., Quan Qi, B., Beasley, S.W. et al.Abnormal branching and regression of the notochord and its relationship to foregut abnormalities. *Eur J Pediatr* Surg 2002;12(2):83-89
10. Arsic, D., Qi, B.Q. and Beasley, S.W Hedgehog in the human: a possible explanation for the VATER association . *J Pediatr Child Health* 2002;38(2):117-121
11. Kluth, D. and Fiegel, D.H. The embryology of the foregut. *Semin Pediatr Surg* 2003;12:3-9
12. Spilde, T.L. Oesophageal atresia: Past, present and future. *J Pediatr Surg* 1996;31:19

13. Spilde, T.L., Bhatia, A.M, Mehta, S. et al. A role for sonic hedgehog signaling in the pathogenesis of human TOF. *J Pediatr Surg* 2003;38:465

14. Vogt, E.C. Congenital atresia of the oesophagus. *AJR Am J Roentgenol* 1929;22:463

15. Gross, R.E. *The Surgery of Infancy and Childhood.* Philadelphia, WB Saunders, 1953.

16. Holder, T.M., Cloud D.T., Lewis J.E. et al. Oesophageal atresia and TOF: A survey of its members by the surgical section of the American Academy of Pediatrics. *Pediatrics* 1964;34:542

17. Shulman, A., Mazkereth, R., Zalel,Y. et al. Prenatal identification of oesophageal atresia: the role of ultrasonography for evaluation of functional anatomy. *Prenat Diagn* 2002;22(8):669-674

18. Beasley, S.W., Allen, M. and Myers, N. The effects of Down syndrome and other chromosomal abnormalities on survival and management in oesophageal atresia. *Pediatr Surg Int* 1997;12(8):550-551

19. Waterston, D.J., Carter, R. and Aberdeen, E. . Oesophageal atresia: Tracheo-oesophageal fistula. A study of survival in 218 infants. *Lancet* 1962;1:819

20. Spitz, L., Kiely, E.M., Morecroft, J. A. Oesophageal atresia: At-risk groups for the 1990s . *J Pediatr Surg* 1994;29:723

21. Iuchtman, M., Brereton R., Spitz L. et al. Morbitity and mortality in 46 patients with the VACTERL association. *Isr J Med* Sci 1992;28:281

22. Foker, J.E., Linden B.C., Boyle Jr. E.M., et al. development of a true primary repair for the full spectrum of oesophageal atresia. *Ann Surg* 1997;226:533

23. Tamburri, N., Laje P., Boglione M. et al. Extrathoracic esophageal elongation (Kimura's technique): a feasible option for the treatment of patients with complex esophageal atresia *Journal of Pediatric Surgery* vol. 44 issue 12 December, 2009. p. 2420-2425

24. Maoate, K., Myers, N.A. and Beasley, S.W. Gastric perforation in infants with oesophageal atresia and distal TOF. *Pediatr Surg Int.* 1999;15(1):24-27

25. Choudhury, S.R., Ashcraft, K.W. and Sharp, R.J. Survival of patients with oesophageal atresia: influence of birth weight, cardiac anomaly, and late respiratory complications. *J Pediatr Surg* 1999;34:70

26. Deurloo, J.A., Ekkelkamp S., Schoorl M. et al. Oesophageal atresia: Histological evolution of management and results in 371 patients. *Ann Thorac Surg* 2002;73:267

27.	Driver, C.P., Shankar, K.R., Jones, M.O. et al. Phenotypic presentation and outcome of oesophageal atresia in the era of Spitz classification. *J Pediatr Surg* 2001;36:1419

28.	Konkin, D.E., O'hali, W.A., Webber E.M. et al. Outcomes in oesophageal atresia and tracheo-oesophageal fistula. *J Pediatr Surg* 2003;38:1726

29.	Orford, J., Cass, D.T. and Glasson, M.J. Advances in the treatment of oesophageal atresia over three decades: the 1970s and the 1990s. *Pediatr Surg Int* 2004;20:402

30.	Adebo, O.A. Oesophageal atresia and trachoe-oesphageal fistuala. Review of a 10 year experience. *West Afr. J Med* 1990; 9(3):164-169

31.	Sharma, A.K., Shekhawat N.S., Agrawal L.D. et al. Oesophageal atresia and tracheo-oesophageal fistula: A review of 25 years experience. *Pediatr Surg Int.* 2000;16:478

32.	Tönz, M., Köhli, S. and Kaiser, G. Oesophageal atresia: What has changed in the last 3 decades? *Pediatr Surg Int* 2004;20:768-772.

Chapter 16
Outcome of Treatment of Clubfoot at the Korle Bu Orthopaedic Unit Using the Ponseti Method

Bandoh, A. K, Addo, A. O, Segbefia, M.

Introduction

Clubfoot is a complex developmental deformation of the foot and the genes responsible for the deformity has been reported to be active from the 12th to the 20th week of foetal life and can last until three to five years of age. [1]

The deformity has four components; equinus at the ankle, varus at the hindfoot, forefoot adductus and cavus. The goal of treatment is to attain a functional, pain-free, plantigrade foot with good mobility.

In the developing world, many of the cases are untreated or poorly treated, leading to a neglected clubfoot. These children undergo extensive corrective surgery later, often with disturbing failures and complications.The foot after surgery looks better, but is stiff, weak and often painful. Clubfoot in an otherwise normal child can be corrected in two months or less with the Ponseti method of manipulations and plaster cast application with minimal or no surgery. The Ponseti method of correction of clubfoot deformity requires serial corrective casts with long-term brace maintainance of correction. Treatment needs to be started as soon as possible and should be followed under close supervision. [2]

Brace should be worn full-time (day and night) for the first three months after the tenotomy cast is removed, then for 12 hours at night and 2 to 4 hours in the middle of the day, for a total of 14-16 hours (night and naps protocol) during each 24-hour period. In the brace, the knees are left free. Bracing is continued for up to four years of age and the outcomes are good. Morcuende et al.[3] reported a 6 percent relapse rate in compliant patients and 80 percent in non-compliant patients.

This method is suited for developing countries with scarce resources and can be learnt by allied health professionals very easily.[4] The outcomes can be evaluated using the Pirani score which is easy to use with a good interobserver and intraobserver reliability[5] Considering that about 100,000 babies are born worldwide each year, with 80 percent with clubfoot occurring in developing nations,[4] it is important for many more people to learn the Ponseti method. If the clubfoot is not treated, it leads to severe disability where shoe wearing and mobilization are greatly impaired. The deformity associated with the neglected clubfoot is not acceptable and the children often end up receiving extensive surgical procedures resulting in a chronically painful foot.

The current method of early treatment in Ghana is the Ponseti method. Even though the method has been in use for some time, to date, there is no published work on its effectiveness to provide evidence-based prognostic outcome that can inform clinical management of cases. This also makes it difficult to advisee parents and relations on how many casts are required to correct the clubfoot deformity based on the Pirani score

This study provides baseline data on the condition to enable clinicians to manage clubfoot cases adequately and non-operatively and give advice to parents and/or relations on the prognosis of the deformity.

Literature Review

Clubfoot is the commonest congenital deformity in babies. More than 100,000 babies are born worldwide each year with congenital clubfoot. Around 80 percent of the cases occur in developing nations.[4] The male-to-female ratio is high at 3:1.[5] Palmer[6] explained this by suggesting that females require a greater number of predisposing factors than males to produce a clubfoot deformity. Social bias and increased attention towards males in our region can account for the higher incidence in males. The order of birth also seems to have an influence on the occurrence of clubfoot, with 65percent of cases in first-born children, which is in accordance with various studies.[7] There is no relationship of clubfoot to the type of birth.[4]

Many different clubfoot classification systems have been proposed but no single one is universally accepted. At a minimum, a useful classification should distinguish postural, self-resolving clubfoot from true clubfoot which requires orthopaedic treatment. A more advanced classification could discern subtypes of nonsyndromic clubfeet such as complex idiopathic or neurogenic-type clubfeet.[8] An ideal classification would accurately portray the initial severity of the deformity and have prognostic ability.[9] The Pirani score is easy to use and based on physical examination findings. There is excellent interobserver and intraobserver reliability with this scoring system.[10]

Catterall/Pirani (Normal:0 points; most abnormal: 1.0 points)

Hindfoot contracture (HFC)	Points	Midfoot contracture (MFC)	Points
Posterior crease:0,0.5,or 1.0 points		Curvature of lateral border: 0, 0.5,or 1.0 points	
Empty heel:0,0.5,or 1.0 points		Medial crease: 0, 0.5, or 1.0 points	
Rigid equinus:0,0.5, or 1.0 points		c.Lateral head of talus: 0, 0.5, or1.0 points	
HFCS Sub-total		MFCS Sub-total	Total Score(HFCS and MFCS)

The Ponseti method for correcting clubfoot non-operatively has existed for 50 years. The method is especially important in developing countries, where operative facilities are not readily available in the remote areas and few well-trained physicians and personnel can manage the cases effectively with cast treatment only.

There is nearly global agreement that the initial treatment of idiopathic congenital clubfoot should be non-operative, regardless of the severity of the deformity, and should be started as soon as possible after birth.

Ippolito et al.[11] found that the long-term functional results for the Ponseti group were better than those for patients managed with surgery.

A foot scoring 4 or more is likely to require at least four casts, and one scoring less than 4 will require three or fewer. A foot with hindfoot score of 2.5 or 3 has a 72 percent chance of requiring a tenotomy.[10]

The Ponseti method of conservative clubfoot treatment is an excellent method of treatment, of which there have been successful results in the Western countries.[2] The follow-up of patients treated with this deformity has been over 40 years in some studies and these persons are leading a normal adult life. It avoids the complications of surgery and gives a painless, mobile, normal-looking, functional foot which requires no special shoes and allows fairly good mobility. Results of the clubfoot treatment by the Ponseti technique have been good and rewarding and now most clubfeet are treated by this simple method in developed countries.[4] Herzenberg et al.[5] compared two different casting methods (traditional and Ponseti) and found the Ponseti method to be far superior, decreasing the need for operative intervention. In India, where there is a dearth of proper operative facilities in remote areas, this technique is a very safe, easy, result-oriented, economical method of clubfoot management. A study done showed that managing a good referral by proper education and motivation along with integration into other programmmes improves the outcome not only in terms of age at presentation but also for deformity correction. Proper motivation and persuading the parents to accept long-term brace treatment helps maintain the correction over a longer period of time and prevents relapse. Although perfect anatomical or radiographical correction is not achieved, a functional foot is created that lasts for decades.[7]

Methodology

Patients who attended the orthopaedic clinic at the Korle Bu teaching hospital from 2009 until January 2011 were recruited into the study.

This unit receives referrals from the whole country and provides Trauma and Orthopaedic care for patients 24 hours a day, seven days a week. Outpatient clinics for clubfoot management are done twice a week. Approximately 20 clubfoot patients are seen weekly with about three patients being new cases.

A structured questionnaire including a checklist was used to collect data.

Inclusion Criteria

All the patients who were seen during the study period were willing to take part.

Exclusion Criteria

1.   Patients with neglected clubfeet. These are patients who never had any treatment within first 2 years of age.
2.   Recurrent clubfeet. These are patients who developed recurrence after Ponseti treatment of their deformity.
3.   Syndromic clubfeet.

Methodology

The families of selected subjects were contacted and provided with an information sheet while an informed consent was obtained for their children to participate in the study. A pre-tested structured questionnaire was administered to each of the enrolled subjects to document their demographic characteristics as well as the family history where affected relatives were known. The Pirani score was used to evaluate the clubfoot deformity at every two-weekly visit and documented. From the initial score and associated problems of other joints and other deformities, the clubfoot could be classified into idiopathic, postural, and syndromic at the start of treatment. The Ponseti technique was the treatment used.[2] The foot was manipulated to the point where a maximum correction for that visit was attained and held in place by a plaster of Paris cast. At every visit, the cast was removed and the foot evaluated using the Pirani score. It was essential during manipulation to first dorsiflex the first ray of the foot. This seemed to worsen the supination of the foot. The foot was then abducted to correct the adduction. By doing this the calcaneus moved from varus to valgus. Thumb pressure was maintained over the head of the talus and at no time was the thumb placed on the calcaneus. The equinus was the last to be corrected. Tenotomy was sometimes done. Before performing tenotomy, it was assured that the foot was sufficiently abducted. Just before tenotomy, the brace measurements were taken so that by the time the patient was to be fitted with the brace it was ready. The end of cast treatment was determined when after the last cast, at least 30 degrees of passive dorsiflexion was possible, the foot was well corrected, and the operative (tenotomy) scar was minimal. A Steenbeek brace was applied immediately after the last cast was removed, three weeks after tenotomy. For unilateral cases, the brace was set at 70 degrees of external rotation on the clubfoot side, and 40 degrees on the normal side. In bilateral cases, it was set at 70 degrees of external rotation on each side. The bar was of sufficient length so the heels of the shoes were at shoulder width. The bar was bent 5-10 degrees with the convexity away from the child, to hold the feet in dorsiflexion. The child was reviewed as scheduled for complications of casting and compliance.

Data Handling/Statistics

The data were entered into MS Excel and analyzed statistically using SPSS Version 16.0. For continuous socio-demographic data, summary tables of mean, standard deviations and ranges were presented. Chi-square test was used to compare categorical variables. T-test and ANOVA were used to compare means of continuous variables. Correlation analysis was used to establish linear association between scores and duration of treatment as well as number of casts required.

Results and Analysis

A total of 135 patients were recruited for the study over the period. Using the exclusion criteria, 74 patients were analyzed.

There were more males than females in the sample population. Of the total number used for the study 42 percent were females and 58 percent were males.

The correlation graphs show that the rate of drop of score which corresponds to the rate of improvement of the conditions was fastest within the first 6 weeks followed by the tenth week and lowest by the sixteenth week. (*Figures 16.1, 16.2 and 16.3*)

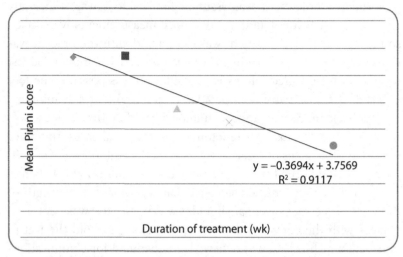

Figure 16.1: Relationship between total score and duration of treatment within first 6 weeks

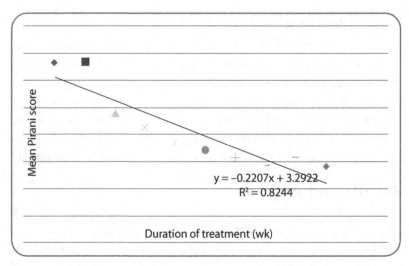

Figure 16.2: Relationship between total score and duration of treatment for 10 weeks

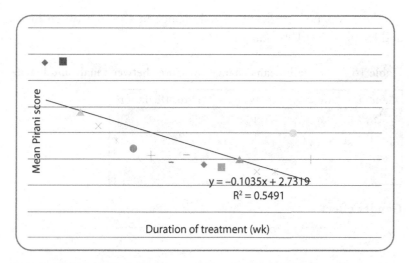

$$y = -0.1035x + 2.7319$$
$$R^2 = 0.5491$$

Duration of treatment (wk)

Figure 16.3: Relationship between total score and duration of treatment for 16 weeks

There was significant correlation between Pirani scores and the duration of treatment at weeks 6, 10 and 16. The highest rate of drop in the scores occurred within the first 6 weeks.
(*Figures 16.1, 16.2 and 16.3*)

There was a steeper drop in Pirani scores for males than for the females. The gradient for the males is -0.203 and -0.097 (*Table 16.1*) for females.

Table 16.1 Correlation coefficients of Pirani scores and duration of treatment

Duration (weeks)	Mean total scores	R^2	Correlation coefficient	p-value	Rate of change in scores /wk
6	2.5	0.9117	-0.955	0.0004	-0.3694
10	2.1	0.8244	-0.908	0.00001	-0.2207
16	1.9	0.5490	-0.741	0.00001	-0.1035

There was no significant overall change in scores between males and females. P=0.106 (*Table 16.2*)

Table 16.2 Overall means changes in scores between male and female

Gender	Mean	N	Std. Deviation
Male	1.6	14	.90
Female	2.0	15	.58
Total	1.8	29	.77

Gender effect

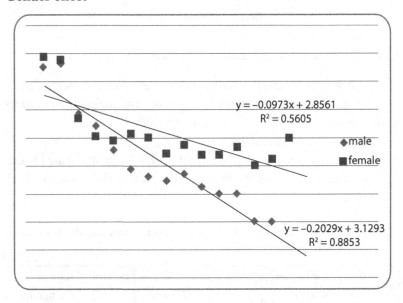

$$y = -0.0973x + 2.8561$$
$$R^2 = 0.5605$$

◆male
■female

$$y = -0.2029x + 3.1293$$
$$R^2 = 0.8853$$

Figure 16.4: Correlation between Pirani scores and duration of treatment for males and females

Majority of the children at presentation had Pirani scores between 1.5 and 2.0 with a few above 2.5 (Figure 16.5)

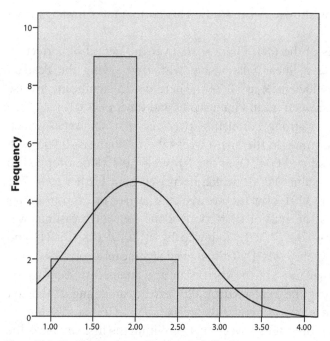

Figure 16.5: Distribution of mean Pirani score of all patients

Table 16.3 **Summary of number of casts**

Mean	3.4
Standard Deviation	1.7
Minimum	1.0
Maximum	8.0
Count	74.0

Discussion

Clubfoot or congenital talipes equinovarus is a complex deformity of the foot that requires meticulous and dedicated efforts on the part of the treating physician and the parent of the child for the correction of the deformity.

This study confirms that the Ponseti method is an effective, reliable method of treating idiopathic clubfeet with good long-term results in Ghanaians. When started early, its outcome can be predicted with the

Pirani score as shown in the study. This corroborates findings from other studies [10]

The means of the total Pirani score over the period of correction was plotted as a linear relationship with time giving the Pearson correlation coefficient R as -0.741. There was a significant inverse relationship between mean Pirani scores and time, p=0001.

There was a strong correlation over the first six weeks which decreased over time. In the first 6 weeks the r value was -0.955 with significant p-value 0.004. Over the 10 weeks, the value dropped to -0.908 with p-value 0.0001 which decreased even further to -0.741 with p-value 0.0001 over the 16 weeks. The rate of drop in scores which implies the rate of correction of the foot after casting, was greatest at 6 weeks (0.369), followed by at 10 weeks (0.221) and finally at 16 weeks (0.104). This showed significant drops, p<0.005. This means that most of the correction was attained in the first six weeks. This may be explained by the better remodeling of the soft tissues influenced by hormones like relaxin on the feet at this time.

The mean score after six weeks is 1.8. Within the first six weeks the number of casts was 3. Out of 74 cases 34 (45.9%) had mean score less than 1.8. Nearly half of the cases would had corrected within the first six week after about 3 casts.

There was significant correlation between means, Pirani scores and number of casts required, r=0.824, p=0.0001. Comparing the r values to the study done by Dyer et al.[10], there was a similar strong correlation coefficient of the study = 0.72 between the Pirani score and the number of casts needed for final correction. The mean number of casts required over the 16-week period was 3 compared to 3.63 by Dyer et al. [10]

This study shows that the Pirani scoring system can be used to estimate the number of weeks of plaster casting required to correct an idiopathic clubfoot.

The initial Pirani scores for patient who had tenotomy ranged from 1.4 to 4.5, with mean score of 3.2 and standard deviation of 1.1. This data is insufficient to predict whether or not a patient may need tenotomy based on his/her initial Pirani score.

The number of children needing tenotomy in our study was 8 percent. In some reports approximately 90 percent of children undergoing Ponseti treatment need a tenotomy.[5] In the Dyer et al.[10] study, the proportion requiring tenotomy was 60 percent. The low need for tenotomy in our study may be due to a better casting technique or high threshold of the surgeon for tenotomy.

There were more males 43 (58 percent) than females 31(42 percent) in our study. The gradient for the regression line for males was -0.203 and for females -0.097. This showed that the deformity correction in males was better than females with clubfoot. The difference however, was not significant, P=0.106

Conclusion

The Ponseti method is an effective method for treating idiopathic clubfeet. When started early after birth, its outcome can be predicted with the Pirani score as shown in the study. Most of the correction takes place in the first six weeks of casting. One cannot predict from the initial score which children would need a tenotomy. The Ponseti method is very cost effective with excellent results and is recommended for widespread use in developing countries.

Limitation

Weekly serial casting as described by Ponseti could not be followed because of the large number of patients seen at the outpatient clinic in addition to the patients with clubfeet. The method was done at a two- weekly interval.

References

1. Cowell, H.R. and Wein, B.K. Genetic aspect of clubfoot. *J Bone Joint Surg Am.* 1980; 62 (8): 1381-1384
2. Ponseti, I.V. Clubfoot management. *J Pediatr Orthop.* 2000; 20(6): 699-700

3. Morcuende, J.A., Dolan, L.A., Dietz, F.R. and Ponseti, I.V. Radical reduction in the rate of extensive corrective surgery for clubfoot using the Ponseti method. *J Pediatr Orthop*. 2004; 113(2):376-380

4. Gupta, A., Singh, S., Patel, P. and Patel, J. Evaluation of the utility of the Ponseti method of correction of clubfoot deformity in a developing nation. *Int. Orthop*. 2008; 32(1): 75-79

5. Herzenberg, J.E., Radler, C. and Bor, N. versus traditional methods of casting for idiopathic clubfoot. *J PediatrOrthop*. 2002; 22:517-21

6. Palmer, R.M. Genetics of talipes equinovarus. *J Bone Joint Surg. Am* .1964; 46:542-556

7. Cooper DM, Dietz FR. Treatment of idiopathic clubfoot: a thirty- year follow-up note. J Bone Joint Surg Am. 1995; 77(10):1477-1489

8. Edmonds, E.W. and Frick, SL. The drop toe sign:an indicator of neurologic impairment in clubfoot. *ClinorthopRelat Res*. 2009; 467:1238-1242.

9. Simons, G.W. *The clubfoot: The present and a view of the Future*. New York: Springer-Verlag;1004

10. Dyer, P.J. and Davis, N . The role of the Pirani scoring system in the management of clubfoot by the Ponseti method. *JBJS Br*. 2006; 88-B:1082-4

11. Ippolito, E., Farsetti, P., Caterini, R. and Tudisco, C. Longterm comparative results in patients with congenital clubfoot treated with two different protocols, *JBJS. Am*. 2003; 85 (7) : 1286-1294

12. Flynn, J., Donohoe, M. and Mackenzie, W.G. An independent assessment of two clubfoot-classification systems. *J PaediatrOrthop*.1998; 18:325-327

13. Chu, A. et al. Clubfoot classification: correlation with Ponseti cast treatment. *J PaediatrOrthop*.2010;**30** (7) 695-699

Chapter 17
Noise Pollution at Work Place and Health Implications

E.D. Kitcher

Introduction

Noise has been the commonest environmental pollutant at industrial workplaces since the industrial revolution. Noise pollution is on the increase due to population growth, urbanization and greater use of mobile sources of sound due to technological advancement. Governmental controls of noise exposure are necessary to protect citizens against the harmful effects of noise. Ancient Rome managed noise pollution at night by banning chariots on roads at night; again measures were also taken in medieval Europe to reduce noise by banning horse-drawn carriages from its streets at night.[1]

Our roads are filled with vehicles which add to noise pollution; furthermore our social activities such as funeral gatherings, wedding receptions and church activities contribute to noise pollution. Our hearing mechanisms are always "on" even when we are asleep.[2] The well-known health consequence of uncontrolled noise pollution at work-place is noise-induced hearing loss.

Noise-induced hearing loss (NIHL) is an irreversible sensorineural hearing loss associated with excessive noise exposure. Noise in excess of 85 dB (A) in a work environment of an eight-hour daily work regime predisposes workers to NIHL.[3] NIHL is usually bilateral and symmetrical, affecting higher frequencies (3k, 4k or 6k Hz) and subsequently lower frequencies (0.5k, 1k or 2k Hz).[4] The global estimates of disabling hearing loss from work-place noice pollution range from 7 percent to 21 percent.[5]

A World Health Organization (WHO) working group concluded that noise is a major threat to human well-being. This article seeks to focus on the local and sub regional experience of the problem of occupational hearing loss. Hearing impairment is defined in relation to hearing thresholds as assessed by pure tone audiometry. Hearing impairment was classified according to the WHO definition;[6] normal hearing < 25 dB hearing threshold level (HTL), mild hearing loss = 26-40 dB HTL, moderate hearing impairment = 41-60 HTL and severe hearing impairment = 61-80dB HTL. The extent of damage to the hearing apparatus is related to duration of exposure and level of intensity of workplace noise levels.[7] Occupational hearing loss may be accompanied by tinnitus, intolerance of loud noise (recruitment) and distortion of perceived sound. The consequence of severe hearing impairment include depression, impaired speech discrimination, impaired job performance, limited job opportunities and sense of isolation.[8, 9, 10]

Methodology

This is a review of articles on noise-induced hearing loss (NIHL) in the sub- region of West Africa. Available literature on NIHL from local workers in the sub-region was obtained from Pubmed and other sources. For this review, a selection was made of articles on comparative studies of evaluation of workers exposed to excessive noise.

The prevalence of NIHL was obtained. These investigators evaluated NIHL of workers in the large scale formal sector and also in the small -scale private sector which is largely unregulated.

Results

Boateng and Amedofu[11] confirmed the presence of noise-induced hearing loss among local sawmills workers with a prevalence of 20 percent, printing press and cornmill workers with prevalence of 7.9 percent and 23 percent respectively. Other local studies by the same authors and others [12] documented the problem of occupational hearing loss among surface gold mining workers with a prevalence of 20 percent. Omokhodion et al[13] noted a prevalence of 56 percent amongst market mill workers. Kitcher et al.[14] noted a prevalence of early occupational hearing loss of 21 percent amongst workers of stone-crushing industry. Ologe et al.[15] in a repeat surveillance for

NIHL amongst bottling factory workers noted a deterioration of hearing amongst these workers and recommended serial audiometry as a means of monitoring deterioration.

McCulllagh et al.[16] in a study of prevalence of hearing loss and accuracy of self-reporting among factory workers noted poor relationship between self-reported hearing ability and the results of audiometry and advocated the need for hearing conservation programmes even in regulated work environments.

It was commonly observed that most workers who were exposed to excessive noise at workplace did not use hearing protection devices even though the noise levels of the work environment was above the normal permissible level of 85dBA.

Discussion

This study confirmed a high prevalence of noise-induced hearing loss. Furthermore most of these workers did not use hearing protection devices due to ignorance or lack of regulation. Some of these industries may not offer regular hearing evaluation of its workers in order to facilitate early detection of NIHL. The high prevalence of occupational hearing loss can be reduced by governmental regulation of work environment through the environmental protection authority and allied bodies. The measures to mitigate exposure to excessive workplace noise pollution will include the compulsory use of hearing protection devices such as ear plugs, and ear muffs. Literature in Ghana, however, confirmed the lack of use of these devices either due to ignorance, or to the discomfort workers felt when wearing them.[17] Furthermore, the availability of hearing protection devices does not automatically lead to regular use by workers.[18] These workers will need to be motivated to use these devices regularly.

Conclusion

There is a high prevalence of occupational hearing loss. Prevention of this health problem includes regulation of the work environment and the enforcement of use of hearing protection devices.

References

1.	Berglund, B. and Lindvall, T. (Eds). *Community Noise. Archives of the Center for Sensory Research.* 1995; 2: 1-195. This document is an updated version of the document published by the World Health Organization in 1995.

2.	Babisch, W. Noise and Health. *Environ Health Perspect* 2005; 113: A14-15.

3.	Rabinowitz, P. and Rees, T. *Textbook of occupational andenvironmental medicine.* 2nd ed. Philadelphia: Elsevier Saunders; 2005. p. 426-36.

4.	National Institute of Health. Consensus conference. Noise and hearing loss. *JAMA* 1990;263:3185-90.

5.	Nelson, D.L., Nelson, R.Y., Concha-Barrientos, M. and Fingeruhut, M. The global burden of occupational noise-induced hearing loss. *Am J Ind Med* 2005;48:446-58.

6.	World Health Organization. Report of the Informal Working Group on Prevention of Deafness and Hearing Impairment, Programme Planning,WHO/PDH/91.1: Geneva:WHO: June 1991. p. 18-21.

7.	Dube, K.J., Ingale, L.T. and Ingale, S.T. Hearing impairement among workers exposed to excessive level of noise in ginning industries. *Noise Health* 2011;13:348-365.

8.	Suter, A.H. Noise and its Effects. Administrative Conference of the United States, 1991. Available at http://www.nonoise.org/library/suter/suter.htm. Accessed: October 10, 2006.

9.	Brookhouser, P. E. Sensorineural hearing loss in children. *Ped Clin N Amer* 1996; 43: 1195-1216.

10.	U.S. Department of Health and Human Services, Public Health Service. *Healthy People 2000: National Health Promotion and Disease Prevention Objectives.* Washington, DC. U.S. Government Printing Office, 1990.

11.	Boating, C. A. and Amedofu, G.K. Industrial noise pollution and its effect on the hearing capabilities of workers: A study from saw mills, printing presses and corn mills. *Afr J Health Sci* 2004;11:55-60.

12.	Amedofu, G.K. Hearing-impairment among workers in a surface gold mining company in Ghana. *Afr J Health Sci* 2002;9:91-7.

13.	Omokhodion, F. O., Adeosun, A. A. and Fajola, A. A. Hearing impairment among mill workers in small scale enterprises in southwest Nigeria. *Noise Health* 2007;9:75-7.

14.   Kitcher, E.D., Ocansey, G. and Tumpi, D.A. Early occupational hearing loss of workers in a stone crushing industry: Our experience in a developing country. *Noise Health* 2012;13:68-71.

15.   Ologe, F.E., Akande, T.M. and Olajide, T.G. Occupational noise exposure and sensorineural hearing loss among workers of a steel rolling mill. *Eur Arch Otorhinolaryngol* 2006;263:618-21.

16.   McCullagh, M.C., Raymond, D., Kerr, M.J. and Lusk, S.L. Prevalence of hearing loss and accuracy of self report among factory workers. *Noise Health* 2011;13:340-347.

17.   Ologe, F. E., Akande, T. M. and Olajide, T. G. Noise exposure, awareness, attitudes and use of hearing protection in a steel rolling mill in Nigeria. *Occup Med* (London).2005 Sep;55(6):48.

18.   Rashaad, Hanisia M. and Dickinson, D. Hearing protection device usage at a South African gold mine. *Occup Med* (Lond). 2010;60:72-4.

Chapter 18
Conclusion

E.Q. Archampong

The revelation that has emerged from the exercise of preparing this manual is the tremendous information base and the fount of technical expertise currently available in the Department of Surgery. However, the concern that strikes any observer must be the challenges of access to these assets. It is evident that with the exception of the paper on the elimination of childhood blindness, which is the product of an on-going project, most of the contributions have emanated from retrospectively collected data in respect of ad hoc stand-alone studies, without clear evidence of continuity in the immediate future. This can not be a dependable means of building the knowledge base of the Department or the institution as a whole. The situation is the result of the paucity of sustainable research projects with appropriate funding. Clearly, if periodic audit studies can yield so much information, it is exciting to imagine how much could be produced through systematic and comprehensive studies based in the Department.

The outcome of the project on elimination of childhood blindness in Ghana is precise information on the causes (bilateral and unilateral) of childhood blindness in the target populations in the Greater Accra and Eastern regions, and what has been achieved, using the team approach strategy, by way of prevention through scientific presentations, public lectures including radio and television interviews and interventions through drug therapies and operations by surgical teams. The project is now in Phase 2 with collaboration between WHO/Lions Club International and the Ghana government, future interventions are expected to be extended to the rest of the country. The study has emphasized the need for continued advocacy nationally and internationally to ensure availability of funding which is the prerequisite for sustainability.

The two papers on breast lesions are timely, given that breast cancer is the commonest female cancer in Ghana and Africa as a whole.

Evidence has been adduced that global developments in management of breast cancer have led to better patient management in Ghana. These include the use of multidisciplinary teams (MDTs) in the formulation of plans. This constitutes the basis for best practice in the management of the disease. There is evidence for the extent to which these practices are being incorporated in breast cancer management in the two main treatment centres in Ghana.

Unfortunately, mammographic screening has not yet taken root in Ghana because of resource limitation; however, the proposal for clinical breast examination, breast self-examination and opportunistic screening has been strongly recommended. Tripple assessment, i.e. clinical examination, imaging procedures and tissue sampling, remains the basis for diagnosis. The challenge for Ghanaian surgeons currently, is the development of methods for taking a biopsy of non-palpable breast lesions. Advances have been noted in all the treatment modalities i.e. surgery, radiotherapy, chemotherapy and hormone therapy. Biological therapy in the treatment of patients with HER2 receptor over-expression is available but the outcome is often hindered by the high cost of treatment.

It is reassuring that breast cancer management in Ghana has kept pace with global developments. The young age of the breast cancer patient in Ghana, attendant socio-cultural differences and prevailing financial limitations indicate significant modifications in the approach to management of the condition in the country.

The study of benign and pre-malignant breast disease has also revealed significant increase in ductal carcinoma in situ and this carries a higher risk of invasive carcinoma. It should therefore be treated appropriately to prevent this progression to the disease. There is an urgent need for investment in the work of the Breast Cancer Clinic and activities of the MDTs in response to the apparent increased breast cancer incidence in the country.

The papers on acute appendicitis, peptic ulcer disease (and complications), gastrointestinal tumours and obstructive biliary disease all point to the rising incidence of these lifestyle related diseases in the Ghanaian population, and call attention to the need for health education on healthy eating habits, regular exercise and need for stress control in socio-cultural activities. The striking observation from these studies is the close resemblance of the natural history, diagnosis and management of these conditions and their complications to the presentation in Western countries. The principal difference is the poorer outcome of management, which stems from delays in presentation and the prevailing resource limitation in the developing world. There would never be enough resources for all the desirable improvements in diagnosis and management. Research must seriously confront the need to factor resource management into our approach to treatment of these diseases, whatever the intervention – use of antibiotics in appendicitis, use of blood and blood products in peptic ulcers or surgical operations on gastrointestinal cancers.

Lower urinary tract obstruction (LUTO) is a condition produced by several diseases of the urinary tract, but principally prostatic hypertrophy/cancer and urethral stricture, the departmental experience is reviewed in this contribution. There is an effective protocol for the management of the causes of LUTO; the real challenge to satisfactory service to the public derives from resource limitation, which is the reason for the large numbers of otherwise fit men that continue to depend on catheter bladder drainage for years. Prostatic cancer as the second commonest cause of cancer death in the male continues to pose problems for various reasons, foe example, the clinical significance of a raised serum prostatic antigen (PSA) scanning for metastatic disease and resistance to chemotherapy or hormone therapy. The expertise for radical prostatectomy for early cases is now available with an improving learning curve.

The contribution from the Orthopaedic Unit provides convincing evidence-based support for the adoption of a simple, readily applicable regime for the cost-effective management of the common clubfoot deformity. The evidence needs to be expanded through a wider prospective study involving satellite centres affiliated to the Orthopaedic Unit. This is an important departmental development because the principle can be readily applied to the several other limb deformities which swell attendance at the orthopaedic clinics.

The departmental experience of the evolution of a centre of excellence is vividly recounted through the story of the National

Cardiothoracic Centre in the Korle Bu Teaching Hospital complex. . Clearly this has encouraged the government of Ghana to replicate this in other fields of surgery on the compound. It may yet stimulate other developments in the health sector further afield.

One contribution which has wider application beyond the field of surgery and hospital medical practice is the paper from the Ear, Nose and Throat section on noise pollution in the workplace and the environment. The paper highlights the extremely high prevalence of noise-induced hearing loss (NIHL) associated with particular occupational environment: - sawmills, printing press, cornmills, gold mines and the stone-crushing industry. In these places the noise level often exceeds the accepted health level of 85 decibels. Unfortunately, when established, it is an irreversible sensory neural hearing loss with prevalence varying from one occupation to the other, of the order of 20 percent to 56 percent.

Regulation of the work environment by government appointed agencies is crucial to prevention, but health attendants are frustrated by the low use of hearing protection devices provided. Enforced monitoring of hearing impairment in the work place would appear to be the way forward.

This manual has raised some weighty issues which impact on management of surgical problems and other aspects of health care. Regrettably there are notable gaps and omissions in the coverage of essential items and expertise. However, in the process, the stage has been set for the evolution of formal protocols for the management of the conditions presented in this Reader as a guide to standard practice as obtains in the premiere medical centre in Ghana. In essence, this publication cannot be an event, but rather a dynamic process stimulating the production of future Readers under the general theme of Recent Advances in Surgical Practice. This is the way forward.

Index

A

Adenocarcinoma 81, 82, 86, 109, 147, 157

Adenoma
  tubular · 106,108
  tubulo-villous · 106
  villous · 106

Alfuzosin · 155

allied surgery · 1,171

Alpha adrenergic blockers · 155

amoebic colitis · 126

anastomosis · 69, 122, 124, 133, 142, 143, 158, 189, 190

anastomotic stricture · 159

aneurysm · 100,166

angiodysplasias · 89, 118, 128, 131

Anti-angiogenesis ·31

aortic valve · 169

Aorto-Enteric Fistula · 100

Apoptosis · 30, 159, 183, 191

Aromatase Inhibitors · 28-30, 36

artificial heart · 170

atrial septal defect · 168

Avastin · *See* immunotherapy112

B

Balloon tamponade · 97

Barium enema · 56,110

Benign Prostate Hyperplasia
  investigation · 159
  presentation · 171
  treatment · 171

Bicalutamide · 159

Bilroth II 69

Biopsy
  endomyocardial · 170
  transrectal ultrasound-guided ·164
  stereotactic · 23
  bladder calculi · 155, 156, 162

bladder diverticula · 123, 130, 155,162

Blalock-Taussig Shunt · 165,175

Bleeding varices · 175

bleeding oesophageal varices 88, 89, 90, 91, 97

Blindness 5-8, 10-17, 212

Blummer's shelf · 109

brachytherapy · 158,159

Breast cancer
  clinical trials · 12,21,33
  diagnosis of · 21,23
  Multidisciplinary team · 19, 20, 47, 213
  pathology report of · 19, 20, 23, 24, 32, 34, 50
  protocols · 20
  screening for · 3, 21, 22, 32-34, 39, 40
  treatment of
    biological therapy in 32,213
    chemotherapy in 24, 25, 27, 28, 30, 32, 34, 35, 36
    hormonal therapy in 24, 28, 32, 35, 36, 48
    radiotherapy in 19, 24, 25, 31, 32, 35-38
    surgery of axilla in · 24-27, 35, 39, 47, 48
    surgery of breast in · 24,26
    tumour board · 20

Breast self-examination 22,213

C

capsule endoscopy · 117, 127, 129
carcinoembryonic antigen · 110
cardiac catheterization· 166, 167, 171, 173
cardiac failure · 167
cardiac pacemaker · 169, 180
cardiac stimulation · 169
Cardioplegic cardiac arrest · 174
cardiopulmonary perfusion · 171
CEA · 110
Chermotherapy 27, 35, 36
chemoradiation · 81, 84, 111, 116
clinical breast examination 22, 41, 213
CLO test · 66
Colonoscopy 110, 117, 120, 121, 127-130
  CT colonography · 110
  CT pneumocolon · See CT colonography
  Virtual colonoscopy · See CT colonography
Colorectal carcinoma · 106, 108, 109, 113, 115, 116, 118, 122, 125
congenital heart disease · 167, 168, 188
coronary artery disease · 169
cyanotic heart disease · 167
Cyclosporin-A · 170
cystocele · 161,162
Cystoscopy · 162
cystostomy · 150,151
cystourethrogram · 151
Cytostatic · 27, 30, 31
Cytotoxic · 27, 30, 111
cytotoxic chemotherapy
  5-fluorouracil · 111

Capecitabine · 85,111
Irinothecan · 111
Leucovorin · 111
Oxaliplatin · 111

D

da Vinci system · 179
detrusor · 148, 154, 160, 162
detrusor-sphincter-dyssynergia · 149
Diethylstilboesterol · 159
Dieulafoy's Lesions · 89, 99, 127
Digital mammography · 160
Dimercaptosuccinic acid · 160
Diverticular disease · 51, 107, 188, 199, 122, 123, 128-130
DMSA · See
donor · 14, 170, 180
double balloon endoscopy · 117, 127
Dukes stage · 109, 111, 112
dyspepsia · 65, 66, 72, 91, 95, 217

E

electrodes · 169
Elimination of Childhood Blindness Project in Ghana 5, 6, 13, 15, 16, 212
  SWOT Analysis · 13
empyema · 166
endocytosis ·31
endometriomata · 108
endoscopic treatment 96, 97, 102
  ligation · 96, 97, 99, 103, 120, 125, 132
  sclerotherapy · 96, 97, 103, 125

W

Z

V

Printed in the United States
By Bookmasters